STUDY GUIDE FOR

STRUCTURE & FUNCTION OF THE BODY

Thirteenth Edition

Prepared by

Linda Swisher, RN, EdD

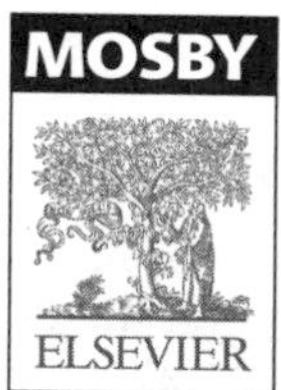

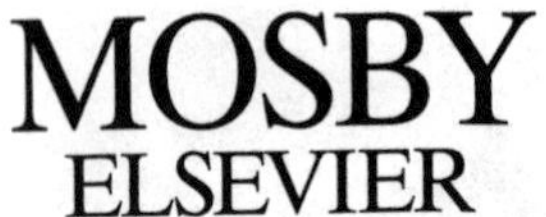

11830 Westline Industrial Drive
St. Louis, Missouri 63146

Study Guide for Structure & Function of the Body

ISBN-13: 978-0-323-04965-8
ISBN-10: 0-323-04965-6

Notice

Neither the Publisher nor the Authors assume any responsibility for any loss or injury and/or damage to persons or property arising out of or related to any use of the material contained in this book. It is the responsibility of the treating practitioner, relying on independent expertise and knowledge of the patient, to determine the best treatment and method of application for the patient.

The Publisher

ISBN-13: 978-0-323-04965-8
ISBN-10: 0-323-04965-6

Managing Editor: Jeff Downing
Developmental Editor: Allison Brock
Publishing Services Manager: Deborah Vogel
Project Manager: Deon Lee
Cover Designer: Kim Denando

Printed in USA
Last digit is the print number: 9 8 7 6 5 4 3 2 1

Preface

TO THE INSTRUCTOR

This study guide is designed to help your students master basic anatomy and physiology. It works in two ways.

First, the section of the preface titled "To the Student" contains detailed information about the following topics:

- How to achieve good grades in anatomy and physiology
- How to read the textbook
- How to use the exercises in this study guide
- How to use visual memory as a learning tool
- How to use mnemonic devices as learning aids
- How to prepare for an examination
- How to take an examination
- How to find out why questions were missed on an examination

Second, the study guide itself contains features that facilitate learning. These features include the following:

1. LEARNING OBJECTIVES, designed to break down the information to be mastered into smaller, more manageable units. The questions in this study guide have been developed to help the student master the learning objectives that are identified at the beginning of each chapter in the text. The guide is also sequenced to correspond to key areas of each chapter. A variety of questions has been prepared to cover the material effectively and to expose the student to several different approaches to learning.
2. CROSSWORD PUZZLES, WORD FINDS, and UNSCRAMBLE THE WORDS to encourage the use of new vocabulary words and emphasize the proper spelling of these terms in an entertaining manner.
3. OPTIONAL APPLICATION QUESTIONS, particularly targeted for the health occupations student but appropriate for any student of anatomy and physiology because they are based entirely on information contained within the chapter.
4. DIAGRAMS, with key features marked by numbers for identification. Students can easily check their work by comparing the diagram in the workbook with the equivalent figure in the text.
5. PAGE NUMBER REFERENCES, found in the "Answers to Chapter Exercises" section. Each answer is cross-referenced with the page in the text where the information supporting that answer is found. Additionally, questions are grouped by specific topics that correspond to sections of the text. Following each major section of the study guide are references to specific areas of the text that will help students who are having difficulty with a particular grouping of questions. These references will point the students to the part of the text on which they should focus their study. These references are of great assistance to both instructor and student because remedial work is made easier and more effective when the area of weakness is identified accurately.
6. ONE LAST QUICK CHECK, found at the end of each chapter. Students can determine how successfully they have retained the information from each section test in the chapter by taking this sample test of questions reviewing all areas of the text.

These features should make mastery of the material contained in this text and study guide a rewarding experience for both instructor and student.

TO THE STUDENT

How to Achieve Good Grades in Anatomy and Physiology

This study guide is designed to help you succeed in learning anatomy and physiology. Before you begin using the study guide, read the following suggestions. Understanding effective study techniques and having good study habits will help you become a more successful student.

How to Read the Textbook

Keep up with the reading assignments. Read the textbook assignment before the instructor covers the material in a lecture. If you have failed to read the assignment beforehand, you will not grasp what the instructor is talking about in lecture. When you read, do the following:

1. As you finish reading a sentence, ask yourself if you understand it. If you do not, put a question mark in the margin by that sentence. If the instructor does not clear up the problem in a lecture, ask him or her to explain it to you.
2. Make sure you can perform all of the learning objectives in the text. A learning objective is a specific task that you are expected to be able to do after you have read a chapter. The objectives set specific goals and break down learning into small steps. They emphasize the key points that the author is making in the chapter.
3. Underline the text and make notes in the margin to highlight key ideas, to mark something you need to reinforce at a later time, or to indicate things that you do not understand.
4. If you come to a word you do not understand, look it up in a dictionary. Write the word on one side of an index card, and write its definition on the other. Carry these cards with you, and when you have a spare minute, use them like flash cards (like you may have done when you were learning your multiplication tables). If you do not know how to spell or pronounce a word, you will have a hard time remembering it.
5. Carefully study each diagram and illustration as you progress through the text. Many students ignore these aids, but the author included them to help you understand the material.
6. Summarize what you read. After you finish a paragraph, try to restate the main ideas. Do this again when you finish the chapter. In your mind, identify and review the main concepts of the chapter, then check to see if you are correct. In short, be an active reader. Do not just stare at a page or read it superficially.

Finally, approach each unit of learning with a positive mental attitude. Motivation and perseverance are prime factors in your effort to achieve successful grades. The combined effects of your instructor, the text, the study guide, and your dedicated work will lead to your success in anatomy and physiology.

How to Use the Exercises in This Study Guide

After you have read a chapter and learned all the new vocabulary it contains, begin working with the study guide. Read the overview of the chapter, which summarizes the main points.

Familiarize yourself with the "Topics for Review" section of the overview, which emphasizes the learning objectives that were outlined in the text. Complete the questions and diagrams in the study guide. The questions have been sequenced to follow the chapter outline and headings, and they are divided into small sections to facilitate learning. A variety of questions is offered throughout the study guide to help you cover the material effectively. The following examples are among the exercises that have been included to assist you.

Multiple Choice Questions

Multiple choice questions will offer you many options to select from, but only one answer will be correct. There are two types of multiple choice questions that you may not be familiar with that have been included in this study guide:

1. "None of the above" questions. These questions test your ability to recall rather than recognize the correct answer. You would select the "none of the above" answer only if all of the other possible answers for a particular question were incorrect.
2. Sequence questions. These questions test your ability to arrange a list of structures in the correct order. In this type of question, you are asked to determine the sequence of structures from the various choices given. An example of this type of question might be the following:

   Which one of the following structures would be the third through which food would pass?
   A. Stomach
   B. Mouth
   C. Large intestine
   D. Esophagus
   E. Anus

   The correct answer would be A.

Matching Questions

Matching questions ask you to select the correct answer from a list of options and to write the answer in the space provided.

True or False Questions

True or false questions ask you to write "T" in the answer space next to a statement if you feel the statement is correct. If you believe the statement to be incorrect, you will circle the word or words that make the statement incorrect and write the correct word or words in the answer blank.

Identify the Term that Does Not Belong

In questions that ask you to identify the term that does not belong, you are given a series of four words. Three words are given that are related to each other in structure or function, and another word is included that has no relationship to, or that has an opposing relationship to, the other three terms. You are to circle the term that does not relate to the other three terms. An example might be the following:

Iris Cornea Stapes Retina

You would circle "Stapes" because all of the other terms refer to parts of the eye.

Fill-in-the-Blank Questions

Fill-in-the-blank questions ask you to make judgments about a situation based on the information presented in the chapter. These questions may ask you how you would respond to a situation or what you would suggest as a possible diagnosis when you are given a set of symptoms.

Charts

Several charts have been included that correspond to figures in the text. Certain areas of these charts have been omitted so that you can fill them in to test your recall of these important areas.

Word Finds

The study guide includes word find puzzles that allow you to identify key terms in the chapter in an interesting and challenging way.

Crossword Puzzles

Vocabulary words from the "New Words" section at the end of each chapter of the text have been developed into crossword puzzles. This format encourages both recall and proper spelling. Occasionally an exercise will include scrambled words. This, too, encourages recall and spelling.

Labeling Exercises

Labeling exercises present diagrams with parts that are not identified. For each of these diagrams, you are to print the name of each numbered part on the corresponding numbered line. You may choose to further distinguish the structures by coloring them with a variety of colors. After you have written down the names of all the structures to be identified, check your answers. When it comes time to review before an examination, you can place a sheet of paper over the answers you have already written on the lines. This procedure will allow you to test yourself a second time without seeing the answers.

After completing the exercises in the study guide, check your answers. If they are not correct, refer to the page listed with the answer and review it for further clarification. If you still do not understand the question or the answer, ask your instructor for further explanation.

If you have difficulty with several questions from one section, refer to the pages given at the end of the section ("If you have had difficulty with this section, review pages...). After reviewing the section, try to answer the questions again. If you are still having difficulty, talk to your instructor.

One Last Quick Check

This exercise, located at the end of each chapter, provides you with an opportunity to test your recall of the entire chapter. A sample test comprised of key material allows you to test your ability to retain the entire chapter after you have mastered all the individual units.

How to Use Visual Memory

Visual memory is another important learning tool. If you were asked to picture in your mind an elephant with all of its external parts labeled, you could do that easily. Visual memory is a powerful key to learning. Whenever possible, try to build a memory picture. Remember, a picture is worth a thousand words.

Visual memory works especially well with the sequencing of items such as circulatory pathways and the passageways of air and food. Students who try to learn sequencing by memorizing a list of words do poorly on examinations. If they forget one word in the sequence, then they will forget all the words after the forgotten one as well. However, if you have a strong memory picture, you will be able pick out the important features even if you have forgotten some of the lesser ones.

How to Use Mnemonic Devices

Mnemonic devices are little jingles that you memorize to help you remember things, particularly items in a sequence. If you make up your own, they will stick with you longer. Here are three examples of such devices:

1. "On Old Olympus' Towering Tops A Finn And German Viewed Some Hops." This mnemonic device is used to remember the order of the 12 pair of cranial nerves. Each word begins with the same letter, as does the name of one of the nerves.
2. "C. Hopkins CaFe where they serve Mg NaCl." This one reminds you of the chemical symbols for the biologically important electrolytes.
3. "Roy G. Biv." A very popular mnemonic device, this one helps you to remember the order of the colors of the visible light spectrum.

How to Prepare for an Examination

Prepare for an examination far in advance. Actually, your preparation for an examination should begin on the first day of class. Keeping up with your daily assignments makes the final preparation for an examination much easier. You should begin your final preparation at least three nights before a test. Last-minute studying usually means poor results and limited retention of the material. The following suggestions may help you improve your test results:

1. Make sure that you understand and can perform all of the learning objectives for the chapter on which you are being tested.
2. Review the appropriate questions in this study guide. Reviewing is something that you should do after every class and at the end of every study session. It is important to keep going over the material until you have a thorough understanding of the chapter and a rapid recall of its contents. If review becomes a daily habit, studying for the actual examination will not be difficult. Go through each question in the study guide and write down an answer. Do the same for the exercises in which you label each structure on a diagram. If you have already done this as part of your daily review, cover the answers with a piece of paper and quiz yourself again.
3. Check the answers that you have written down against the correct answers in the back of the study guide. Go back and study the areas in the text that refer to questions that you answered incorrectly and then try to answer those questions again. If you still cannot answer a question or label a structure correctly, ask your instructor for help.
4. As you read a chapter, ask yourself what questions you would ask if you were writing a test for that unit. You will most likely ask yourself many of the questions that will show up on your examination.
5. Get a good night's sleep before the test. Staying up late and upsetting your biorhythms will only make you less efficient during the test.

How to Take an Examination

The Day of the Test

1. Get up early enough to avoid rushing. Eat appropriately. Your body needs fuel, but a heavy meal just before a test is not a good idea.
2. Keep calm. Briefly look over your notes. If you have properly prepared for the test, there will be no need for last-minute cramming.
3. Make sure that you have everything you need to take the test: pens, pencils, test sheets, and so forth.
4. Allow enough time to get to the examination site. Missing your bus, getting stuck in traffic, or being unable to find a parking space will not put you in a good frame of mind to do well on the examination.

During the Examination

1. Pay careful attention to the instructions for the test.
2. Note any corrections.
3. Budget your time so that you will be able to finish the test.
4. Ask the instructor for clarification if you do not understand a question or an instruction.
5. Concentrate on your own test paper and do not allow yourself to be distracted by others in the room.

Hints for Taking a Multiple Choice Test

1. Read each question carefully. Pay attention to each word.
2. Cross out obviously wrong answers and then carefully consider those that are left.
3. Go through the test once and quickly answer the questions you are sure about; then go back over the test and answer the rest of the questions.
4. Fill in the answer spaces completely and make your marks heavy. Erase completely if you make a mistake.
5. If you must guess, stick with your first hunch. Most often students will change right answers to wrong ones.
6. If you will not be penalized for guessing, do not leave any blanks.

Hints for Taking an Essay Test

1. Budget time for each question.
2. Write legibly and try to spell words correctly.
3. Be concise, complete, and specific. Do not be repetitious or long-winded.
4. Organize your answer in an outline. This will help you to keep your thoughts organized, and it will also help the person who is grading the test.
5. Answer each question as thoroughly as you can, but leave some room for possible additions.

Hints for Taking a Laboratory Practical Examination

Students often have a hard time with this kind of test. Visual memory is very important in this situation. To put it simply, you must be able to identify every structure you have studied. If you are unable to identify a structure, then you will be unable to answer any questions about that structure.

The types of questions that may appear on this sort of examination include the following:

1. Identification of a structure, organ, or feature.
2. Description of the function of a structure, organ, or feature.
3. Description of the sequence in which air flow, passage of food, elimination of urine, etc., occurs.
4. Disease questions. For example: If the kidney, pancreas, liver, etc., fails, what disease will result?

How to Find Out Why Questions Were Missed on an Examination

After the Examination

Go over your test after it has been scored to see what you missed and why you missed it. You can pick up important clues that will help you on future examinations. Ask yourself these questions:

1. Did I miss questions because I did not read them carefully?
2. Did I miss questions because I had gaps in my knowledge?
3. Did I miss questions because I did not understand certain scientific words?
4. Did I miss questions because I did not have a good visual memory of things?

Be sure to go back and learn the things you did not know. Chances are good that these topics will come up on the final examination.

Your grades in other classes will also improve when you apply these study methods to other courses. Learning should be fun. With these helpful hints and this study guide, you should be able to achieve the grades you desire in your anatomy and physiology class. Good luck!

Acknowledgments

I wish to express my appreciation to the staff of Elsevier, Inc., and especially to Tom Wilhelm, Jeff Downing, and Allison Brock. My continued admiration and thanks to Gary Thibodeau and Kevin Patton for another outstanding edition of their text. Your dedication to science education has given countless students an appreciation for the wonderment of the human body, inspired our future scientists, and contributed to the improvement of health care providers. To my family and Brian, my thanks for your love, assistance, and support throughout this project and my life. Finally, this book is dedicated to the memory of my beloved husband Bill—you will always remain the wind beneath my wings.

Linda Swisher, RN, EdD

Contents

CHAPTER 2

Chemistry of Life

Although anatomy can be studied without knowledge of chemistry, it is hard to imagine an understanding of physiology without a basic comprehension of chemical reactions in the body. Trillions of cells make up the various levels of organization in the body. Our health and survival depends upon the proper chemical maintenance in the cytoplasm of our cells.

Chemists use the terms *elements* or *compounds* to describe all of the substances (matter) in and around us. Distinguishing these two terms is the fact that an element cannot be broken down. A compound, on the other hand, is made up of two or more elements and has the ability to be broken down into the elements that form it.

Organic and inorganic compounds are equally important to us. Without organic compounds such as carbohydrates, proteins, and fats, and inorganic compounds such as water, we could not sustain life.

Because we cannot see many of the chemical reactions that take place daily in our bodies, it is sometimes difficult to comprehend the principles involved in initiating them. Chemicals are responsible for directing virtually all of our bodily functions. It is, therefore, important to master the fundamental concepts of chemistry.

TOPICS FOR REVIEW

Before progressing to Chapter 3, you should have an understanding of the basic chemical reactions in the body and the fundamental concepts of biochemistry.

LEVELS OF CHEMICAL ORGANIZATION

Multiple Choice

Select the best answer.

1. Which of the following is *not* a subatomic particle?
   A. Proton
   B. Electron
   C. Isotope
   D. Neutron

2. Electrons move about within certain limits called:
   A. Energy levels
   B. Orbitals
   C. Chemical bonding
   D. Shells

3. The number of protons in the nucleus is an atom's:
   A. Atomic mass
   B. Atomic energy level
   C. Atomic number
   D. None of the above

4. The number of protons and neutrons combined is the atom's:
   A. Atomic mass
   B. Atomic energy level
   C. Orbit
   D. Chemical bonding

5. Which of the following is *not* one of the major elements present in the human body?
   A. Oxygen
   B. Carbon
   C. Nitrogen
   D. Iron

6. Atoms usually unite with each other to form larger chemical units called:
   A. Energy levels
   B. Mass
   C. Molecules
   D. Shells

7. Substances whose molecules have more than one element in them are called:
   A. Compounds
   B. Orbitals
   C. Elements
   D. Neutrons

True or False

In the space provided, write T for true and F for false.

_____ 8. Matter is anything that occupies space and has mass.

_____ 9. In the body, most chemicals are in the form of electrons.

_____ 10. At the core of each atom is a nucleus composed of positively charged protons and negatively charged neutrons.

_____ 11. Orbitals are arranged into energy levels depending on their distance from the nucleus.

_____ 12. The formula for a compound contains symbols for the elements in each molecule.

If you have had difficulty with this section, review pages 23-25.

CHEMICAL BONDING

Multiple Choice

Select the best answer.

13. Ionic bonds are chemical bonds formed by the:
    A. Sharing of electrons between atoms
    B. Donation of protons from one atom to another
    C. Donation of electrons from one atom to another
    D. Acceptance of protons from one atom to another

14. Molecules that form ions when dissolved in water are called:
    A. Covalent bonds
    B. Electrolytes
    C. Isotopes
    D. Ionic bonds

15. When atoms share electrons, a(n) ____________ forms.
    A. Covalent bond
    B. Electrolyte
    C. Ionic bond
    D. Isotope

16. Covalent bonds:
    A. Break apart easily in water
    B. Are not easily broken
    C. Donate electrons
    D. None of the above

17. An example of an ionic bond is:
    A. NaCl
    B. Ca
    C. O
    D. P

18. If a molecule "dissociates" in water, it:
    A. Has taken on additional ions
    B. Has eliminated ions
    C. Separates to form free ions
    D. Forms a covalent bond

If you have had difficulty with this section, review pages 25-27.

INORGANIC CHEMISTRY

Identify each term with its corresponding description or definition.

A. Aqueous solution
B. Water
C. ATP
D. Base
E. Solvent
F. pH
G. Dehydration synthesis
H. Inorganic
I. Weak acid
J. Hydrolysis
K. Strong acid
L. Reactants

_____ 19. A type of compound

_____ 20. Compound most essential to life

_____ 21. Dissolves solutes

_____ 22. Water plus common salt

_____ 23. Reactants combine only after (H) and (O) atoms removed

_____ 24. Combine to form a larger product

_____ 25. The reverse of dehydration synthesis

_____ 26. Yields energy for muscle contraction

_____ 27. Alkaline compound

_____ 28. A measure of the H^+ concentration

_____ 29. Easily dissociates to form H^+ ions

_____ 30. Dissociates very little

If you have had difficulty with this section, review pages 27-31.

ORGANIC CHEMISTRY

Select the best answer.

(A) Carbohydrate (B) Lipid (C) Proteins (D) Nucleic acid

_____ 31. Monosaccharide

_____ 32. Triglyceride

_____ 33. DNA

_____ 34. Cholesterol

_____ 35. Amino acid

_____ 36. Glycogen

_____ 37. Sucrose

_____ 38. Phospholipid

_____ 39. Contains C, O, H, and N

_____ 40. RNA

If you have had difficulty with this section, review pages 31-37.

CHEMISTRY OF LIFE

Fill in the crossword puzzle.

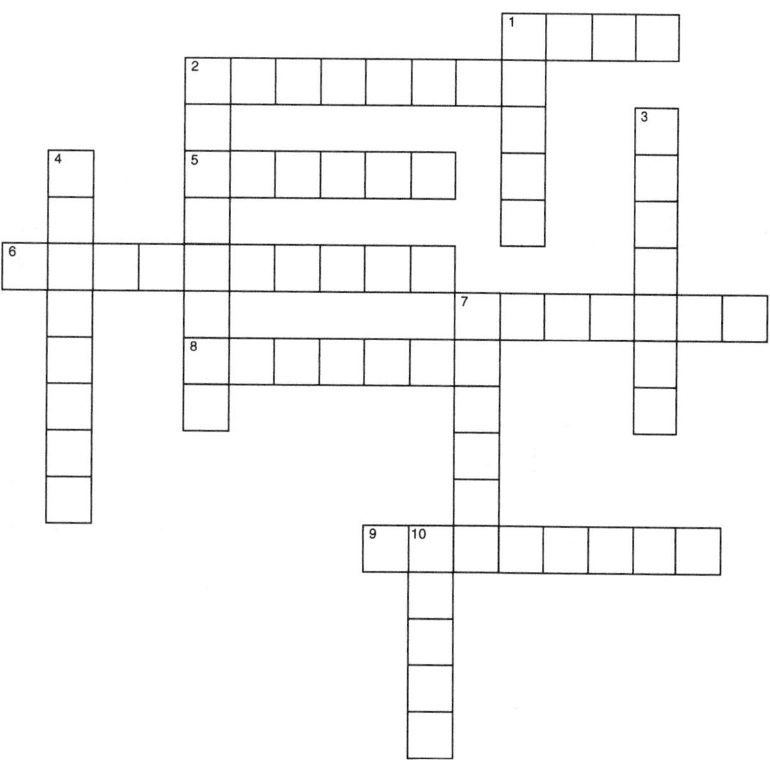

Across

1. Below 7.0 on pH scale
2. Bond formed by sharing electrons
5. Occupies space and has mass
6. Reverse of dehydration synthesis
7. Substances composed of one type of atom
8. Uncharged subatomic particle
9. Subatomic particle

Down

1. Combine to form molecules
2. Substances whose molecules have more than one element
3. Amino acid
4. Polysaccharide
7. Chemical catalyst
10. Fat

UNSCRAMBLE THE WORDS

Take the circled letters, unscramble them, and fill in the statement.

41. **TMATRE**

42. **SETLMENE**

43. **CLSMOEUEL**

44. **NAGRIOC**

45. **RLECETOLYET**

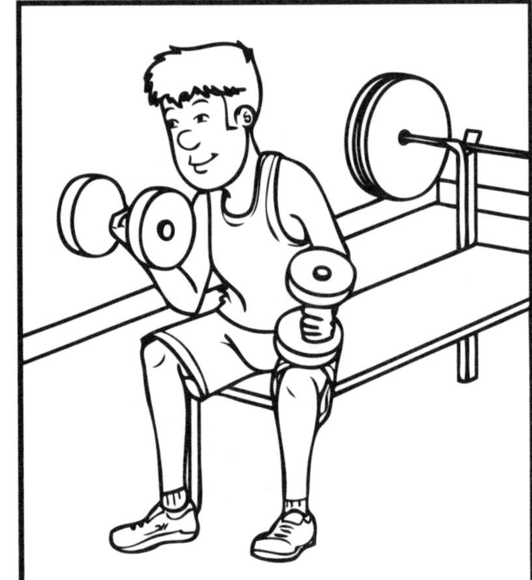

Why Bill worked out each day.

46.

APPLYING WHAT YOU KNOW

47. Sandy just finished preparing a meal of pan-fried hamburgers for her family. While the frying pan was still hot, she poured the liquid grease into a metal container to cool. Later she noticed that the liquid oil had solidified as it cooled. Explain the chemistry of why the now room-temperature fat was solid.

48. Carol was gaining weight, yet she was eating very little. Her physician suspected hypothyroidism and suggested a test that measures radiation emitted by the thyroid when radioactive iodine is introduced into the gland. Describe what the radiologist will do to evaluate Carol's thyroid function.

49. WORD FIND

Can you find 12 terms from this chapter in the box of letters? Words may be spelled top to bottom, bottom to top, right to left, left to right, or diagonally.

Alkaline	Electrolyte
Atomic mass	Molecule
Base	Nucleic acid
Carbohydrate	Proton
Dehydration	Reactant
Dissociation	Solvent

E	T	A	R	D	Y	H	O	B	R	A	C	E
T	B	H	S	I	H	L	I	N	A	T	O	D
B	N	E	H	S	G	O	U	L	P	O	T	E
R	Z	A	M	S	F	R	K	U	S	M	T	H
P	R	O	T	O	N	A	I	E	C	I	X	Y
B	R	N	U	C	L	E	I	C	A	C	I	D
C	A	F	T	I	A	E	W	G	G	M	W	R
L	E	S	N	A	B	E	C	E	E	A	E	A
G	Q	E	E	T	E	A	R	U	S	S	F	T
Q	R	P	V	I	B	Y	K	I	L	S	W	I
E	T	Y	L	O	R	T	C	E	L	E	B	O
S	B	U	O	N	E	S	P	N	B	R	B	N
O	P	J	S	T	D	J	M	O	L	U	H	D

DID YOU KNOW?

After a vigorous workout, your triglycerides fall 10–20% and your HDL increases by the same percentage for 2–3 hours.

When hydrogen burns in the air, water is formed.

CHECK YOUR KNOWLEDGE

Fill in the Blanks

1. ____________________ is the field of science devoted to studying the chemical aspects of life.

2. Atoms are composed of protons, electrons, and ____________________.

3. The farther an orbital extends from the nucleus, the ____________________ its energy level.

4. Substances can be classified as ____________________ or ____________________.

5. Chemical bonds form to make atoms more____________________.

6. A(n) ____________________ is an electrically charged atom.

7. Few ____________________ compounds have carbon atoms in them and none have C-C or C-H bonds.

8. ______________ ____________________ is a reaction in which water is lost from the reactants.

9. Chemists often use a ________________ ____________________ to represent a chemical reaction.

10. High levels of ____________________ in the blood make the blood more acidic.

11. ____________________ are compounds that produce an excess of H^+ ions.

12. ____________________ maintain pH balance by preventing sudden changes in the H^+ ion concentration.

13. ____________________ literally means "carbon" and "water."

14. ____________________ is a steroid lipid.

15. Collagen and keratin are examples of ____________________ proteins.

CHAPTER 3

Cells and Tissues

Cells are the smallest structural units of living things. Therefore, because we are living, we are made up of a mass of cells. Human cells, which vary in shape and size, can only be seen under a microscope. The three main parts of a cell are the cytoplasmic membrane, the cytoplasm, and the nucleus. As you review this chapter, you will be amazed at the resemblance of cells to the body as a whole. You will identify miniature circulatory systems, reproductive systems, digestive systems, power plants (much like muscular systems), and many other structures that will aid in your understanding of these body systems in future chapters.

Cells, just like humans, require water, food, gases, the elimination of wastes, and numerous other substances and processes in order to survive. The movement of these substances into and out of cells is accomplished by two primary methods: passive transport processes and active transport processes. In passive transport processes, no cellular energy is required to effect movement through the cell membrane. However, in active transport processes, cellular energy is required to provide movement through the cell membrane.

The study of cell reproduction completes the chapter's overview of cells. A basic explanation of DNA, "the hereditary molecule," provides a proper respect for the capability of the cell to transmit physical and mental traits from generation to generation. Reproduction of the cell, mitosis, is a complex process requiring several stages. These stages are outlined and diagrammed in the text to facilitate learning.

This chapter concludes with a discussion of tissues that reviews the four main types of tissues: epithelial, connective, muscle, and nervous. Knowledge of the characteristics, location, and function of these tissues is necessary to complete your understanding of the next structural level of organization.

TOPICS FOR REVIEW

Before progressing to Chapter 4, you should have an understanding of the structure and function of the smallest living unit in the body—the cell. Your review should also include the methods by which substances move through the cell membrane and the stages that occur during cell reproduction. As you finish this chapter, you should have an understanding of tonicity and body tissues and the function they perform in the body.

CELLS

Match the term on the left with the proper selection on the right.

Group A

_____ 1. Cytoplasm
_____ 2. Plasma membrane
_____ 3. Cholesterol
_____ 4. Nucleus
_____ 5. Centrioles

A. Component of plasma membrane
B. Controls reproduction of the cell
C. "Living matter"
D. Function in cell reproduction
E. Surrounds and serves as a boundary for cells

Group B

_____ 6. Ribosomes
_____ 7. Endoplasmic reticulum
_____ 8. Mitochondria
_____ 9. Lysosomes
_____ 10. Golgi apparatus

A. "Power plants"
B. "Digestive bags"
C. "Chemical processing and packaging center"
D. "Protein factories"
E. "Smooth and rough"

Fill in the blanks.

11. The numerous small structures that function like organs in a cell are called ____________________.

12. A procedure performed prior to transplanting an organ from one individual to another is ______________ ________________.

13. Fine, hairlike extensions found on the exposed or free surfaces of some cells are called ________________.

14. The process that uses oxygen to break down glucose and other nutrients to release energy required for cellular work is called ________________ or ______________ ______________.

15. ____________________ are usually attached to rough endoplasmic reticulum and produce enzymes and other protein compounds.

16. The ____________________ provide energy-releasing chemical reactions that go on continuously.

17. The organelles that can digest and destroy microbes that invade the cell are called ______________.

18. Mucus is an example of a product manufactured by the ____________.

19. These rod-shaped structures, ______________________, play an important role during cell division.

20. ______________ ______________ are threadlike structures made up of proteins and DNA.

If you have had difficulty with this section, review pages 43-50.

MOVEMENT OF SUBSTANCES THROUGH CELL MEMBRANES

Circle the correct choice.

21. The energy required for active transport processes is obtained from:
    A. ATP
    B. DNA
    C. Diffusion
    D. Osmosis

22. An example of a passive transport process is:
    A. Permease system
    B. Phagocytosis
    C. Pinocytosis
    D. Diffusion

23. Movement of substances from a region of high concentration to a region of low concentration is known as:
    A. Active transport
    B. Passive transport
    C. Cellular energy
    D. Concentration gradient

24. Osmosis is the ____________________ of water across a selectively permeable membrane when some of the solutes cannot cross the membrane.
    A. Filtration
    B. Equilibrium
    C. Active transport
    D. Diffusion

25. ________________________ involves the movement of solutes across a selectively permeable membrane by the process of diffusion.
    A. Osmosis
    B. Filtration
    C. Dialysis
    D. Phagocytosis

26. A specialized example of diffusion is:
    A. Osmosis
    B. Permease system
    C. Filtration
    D. All of the above

27. _______________ always occurs down a hydrostatic pressure gradient.
    A. Osmosis
    B. Filtration
    C. Dialysis
    D. Facilitated diffusion

28. The uphill movement of a substance through a living cell membrane is:
    A. Osmosis
    B. Diffusion
    C. Active transport process
    D. Passive transport process

29. An example of an active transport process is:
    A. Ion pump
    B. Phagocytosis
    C. Pinocytosis
    D. All of the above

30. An example of a cell that uses phagocytosis is the:
    A. White blood cell
    B. Red blood cell
    C. Muscle cell
    D. Bone cell

31. A solution that contains a higher concentration of salt than living red blood cells would be:
    A. Hypotonic
    B. Hypertonic
    C. Isotonic
    D. Homeostatic

32. A red blood cell becomes engorged with water and will eventually lyse, releasing hemoglobin into the solution. This solution is _______________ to the red blood cell.
    A. Hypotonic
    B. Hypertonic
    C. Isotonic
    D. Homeostatic

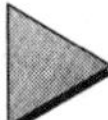
If you have had difficulty with this section, review pages 50-55.

CELL REPRODUCTION

Circle the one that does not *belong.*

33. DNA	Adenine	Uracil	Thymine
34. Complementary	Guanine	Telophase	Cytosinebase pairing
35. Anaphase	Specific sequence	Gene	Base pairs
36. RNA	Ribosome	Thymine	Uracil
37. Translation	Protein synthesis	mRNA	Interphase
38. Cleavage furor	Anaphase	Prophase	2 daughter cells
39. "Resting"	Prophase	Interphase	DNA replication
40. Identical	2 nuclei	Telophase	Metaphase
41. Metaphase	Prophase	Telophase	Gene

If you have had difficulty with this section, review pages 55-59.

50. The nurse was instructed to dissolve a pill in a small amount of liquid medication. As she dropped the capsule into the liquid, she was interrupted by the telephone. On her return to the medication cart, she found the medication completely dissolved and apparently was scattered evenly throughout the liquid. This phenomenon did not surprise her since she was aware from her knowledge of cell transport that _____________________ had created this distribution.

51. Ms. Bence has emphysema. She has been admitted to the hospital and is receiving oxygen per nasal cannula. Emphysema destroys the tiny air sacs in the lungs. These tiny air sacs, called alveoli, provide what function for Ms. Bence?

52. Merrily was 5′4″ and weighed 115 lbs. She appeared very healthy and fit, yet her doctor advised her that she was "overfat." What might be the explanation for this assessment?

53. WORD FIND

Can you find 16 terms from this chapter? Words may be spelled top to bottom, bottom to top, right to left, left to right, or diagonally.

A P D I E V E W N P F E H Y X
I G I Z N S R L X S T W F Z S
R J V N N T A I L M R P H M F
D W U E O O E H B E A D U G F
N W I U I C I R P O N N F B W
O P U R S H Y T P O S A W X K
H X F O U R Y T A H L O G A W
C L Z N F O Y P O R A E M R M
O U I X F M L F O S T S T E O
T T B Y I A B C O T I L E S D
I V S O D T T M I T O S I S U
M N A A I I L E N L N N N F R
E O K K I D C Q H B I V I T H
E K T X B Z A E A L S A E C K
S B Z R P M V L X W Z A Z C V

Chromatid
Cilia
Cuboidal
DNA
Diffusion
Filtration
Hypotonic
Interphase
Mitochondria
Mitosis
Neuron
Organelle
Pinocytosis
Ribosome
Telophase
Translation

DID YOU KNOW?

The largest single cell in the human body is the female sex cell, the ovum. The smallest single cell in the human body is the male sex cell, the sperm.

Other than your brain cells, 50,000,000 of the cells in your body will have died and been replaced with others in the time it took you to read this sentence.

The longest living cells in the body are brain cells, which can live an entire lifetime.

CELLS AND TISSUES

Fill in the crossword puzzle.

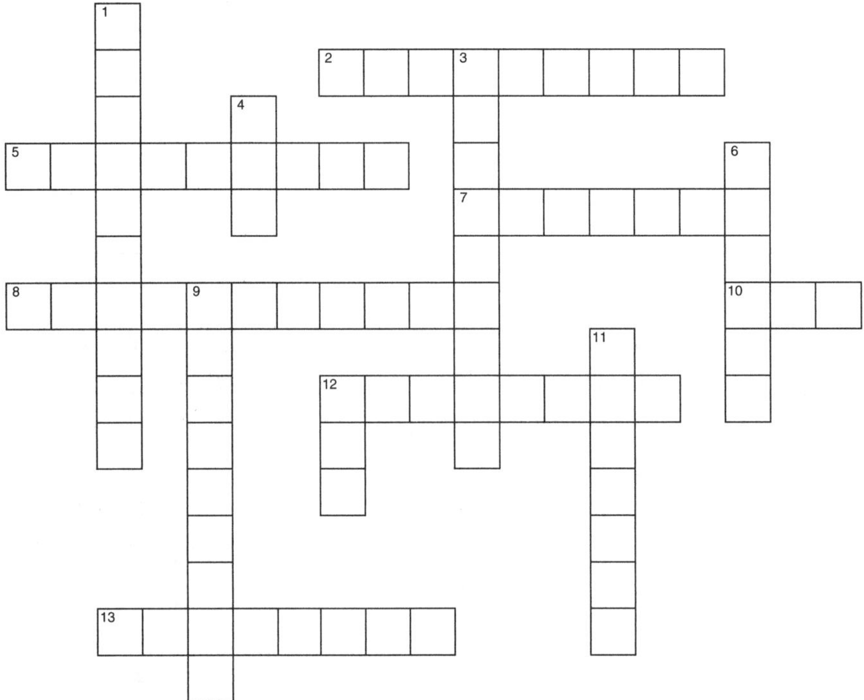

Across
2. Last stage of mitosis
5. Shriveling of cell due to water withdrawal
7. Fat
8. Cartilage cell
10. Ribonucleic acid (abbreviation)
12. Specialized example of diffusion
13. First stage of mitosis

Down
1. Having an osmotic pressure greater than that of the solution with which it is compared
3. Cell organ
4. Energy source for active transport
6. Nerve cell
9. Occurs when substances scatter themselves evenly throughout an available space
11. Reproduction process of most cells
12. Chemical "blueprint" of the body (abbreviation)

CHECK YOUR KNOWLEDGE

Multiple Choice

Circle the correct answer.

1. The internal living material of cells is / are the:
   A. Cytoplasm
   B. Plasma membrane
   C. Nucleus
   D. Centrioles

2. The "protein factories" of the cell are the:
   A. Mitochondria
   B. Ribosomes
   C. Lysosomes
   D. Golgi apparatus

3. The process of enzymes using oxygen to break down glucose and other nutrients to release energy required for cellular work is:
   A. Chemical processing
   B. Cellular respiration
   C. Apoptosis
   D. Passive transport

4. Two of these rod-shaped structures exist in every cell.
   A. Centrioles
   B. Cilia
   C. Ribosomes
   D. Lysosomes

5. Adenosine triphosphate is the chemical substance that provides the energy required for:
   A. Passive transport
   B. Osmosis
   C. Active transport
   D. Dialysis

6. A solution that contains a lower concentration of salt than living red blood cells would be:
   A. Hypotonic
   B. Hypertonic
   C. Isotonic
   D. Homeostatic

7. It is the sequence of base pairs in each gene of each chromosome that determines:
   A. Anaphase
   B. Thymine
   C. Translation
   D. Heredity

8. The specific and visible stages of cell division are preceded by a period called:
   A. Anaphase
   B. Interphase
   C. Prophase
   D. Metaphase

9. Which of the following is *not* an example of muscle tissue?
   A. Smooth
   B. Skeletal
   C. Hemopoietic
   D. Cardiac

10. Stratified squamous epithelium assists the body by providing:
    A. Anchors for our bones
    B. Support for the body
    C. Contractility
    D. Protection against invasion by microorganisms

Matching

Select the most correct answer from column B for each statement in column A. (Only one answer is correct.)

Column A	Column B
_____ 11. Endoplasmic reticulum	A. Phagocytosis
_____ 12. Flagellum	B. 0.9% NaCl solution
_____ 13. Chromosomes	C. Osmosis
_____ 14. Passive transport	D. Cell division complete
_____ 15. Active transport	E. Blood
_____ 16. Isotonic	F. Rough and smooth
_____ 17. Transcription	G. Tail of the sperm cell
_____ 18. Anaphase	H. Cleavage furrow
_____ 19. Telophase	I. Translation
_____ 20. Connective tissue	J. DNA

CELL STRUCTURE

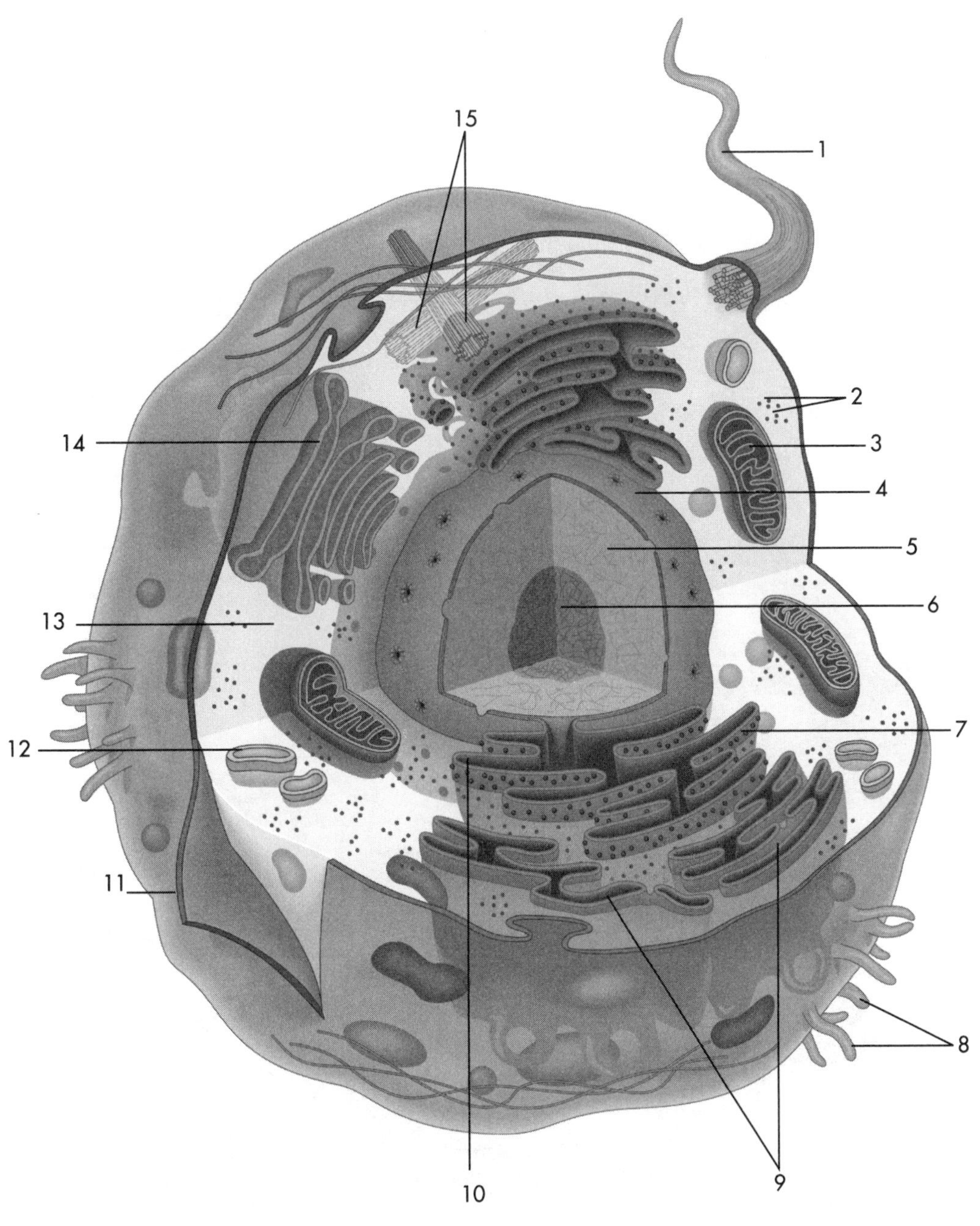

1. ______________________
2. ______________________
3. ______________________
4. ______________________
5. ______________________
6. ______________________
7. ______________________
8. ______________________
9. ______________________
10. ______________________
11. ______________________
12. ______________________
13. ______________________
14. ______________________
15. ______________________

MITOSIS

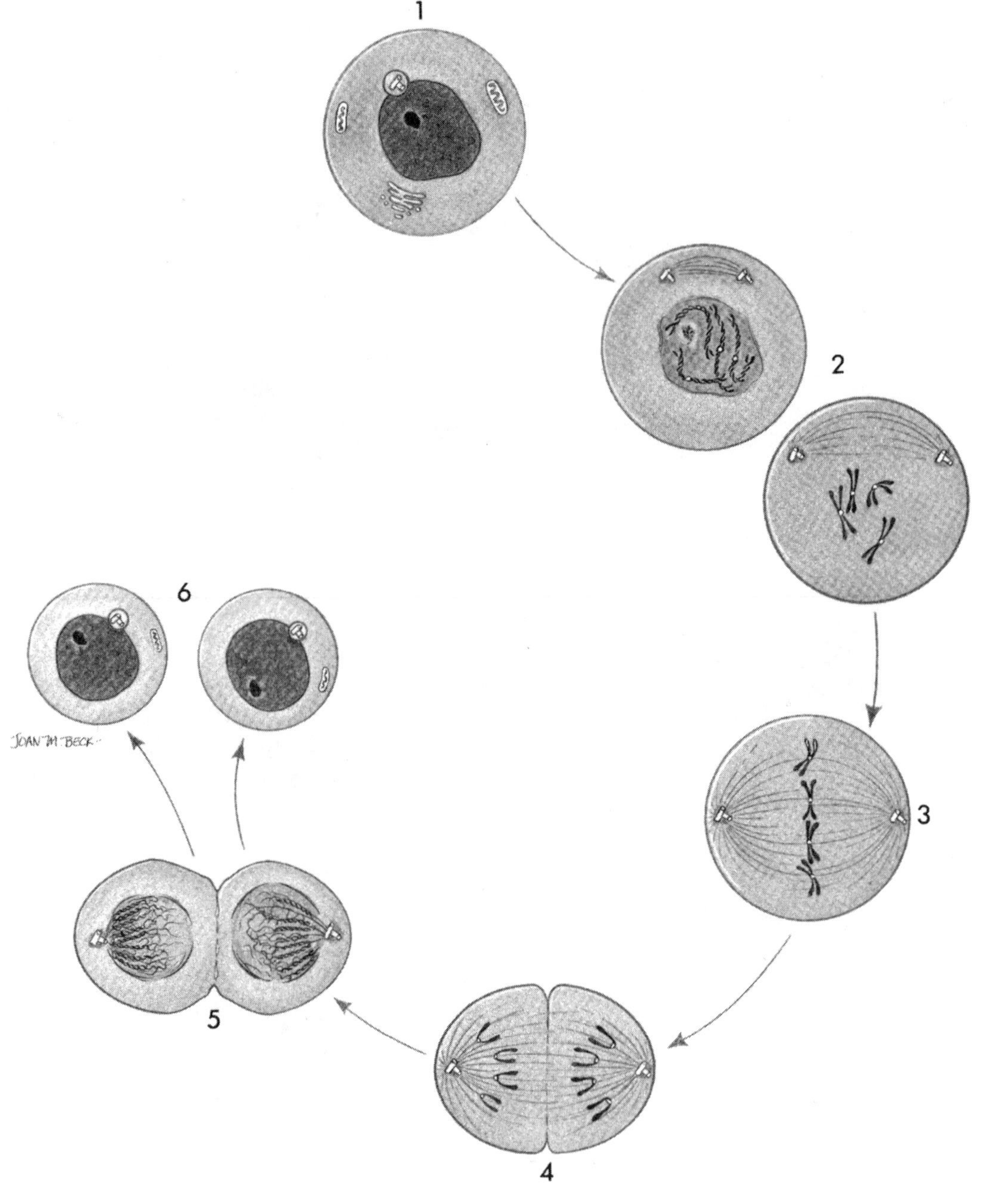

1. ______________________
2. ______________________
3. ______________________
4. ______________________
5. ______________________
6. ______________________

CHAPTER 4

Organ Systems of the Body

A smooth-running automobile is the result of many systems harmoniously working together. The engine, the fuel system, the exhaust system, the brake system, and the cooling system are but a few of the many complex structural units that the automobile as a whole relies on to keep it functioning smoothly. So it is with the human body. We, too, depend on the successful performance of many individual systems working together to create and maintain a healthy human being.

When you have completed your review of the 11 major organ systems and the organs that make up these systems, you will find your understanding of the performance of the body as a whole much more meaningful.

TOPICS FOR REVIEW

Before progressing to Chapter 5, you should have an understanding of the 11 major organ systems and be able to identify the organs that are included in each system.

ORGAN SYSTEMS OF THE BODY

Match the term on the left with the proper selection on the right.

Group A

_____	1. Integumentary	A. Hair
_____	2. Skeletal	B. Spinal cord
_____	3. Muscular	C. Hormones
_____	4. Nervous	D. Tendons
_____	5. Endocrine	E. Joints

Group B

_____	6. Circulatory	A. Esophagus
_____	7. Lymphatic	B. Ureters
_____	8. Urinary	C. Larynx
_____	9. Digestive	D. Genitalia
_____	10. Respiratory	E. Spleen
_____	11. Reproductive	F. Capillaries

Circle the one that does not *belong.*

12. Pharynx	Trachea	Mouth	Alveoli
13. Uterus	Rectum	Gonads	Prostate
14. Veins	Arteries	Heart	Pancreas
15. Pineal	Bladder	Ureters	Urethra
16. Cardiac	Smooth	Joints	Voluntary
17. Pituitary	Brain	Spinal cord	Nerves
18. Cartilage	Joints	Ligaments	Tendons
19. Hormones	Pituitary	Pancreas	Appendix
20. Thymus	Nails	Hair	Oil glands
21. Esophagus	Pharynx	Mouth	Trachea
22. Thymus	Spleen	Tonsils	Liver

Fill in the missing areas.

SYSTEM	ORGANS	FUNCTION
23. Integumentary	Skin, nails, hair, sense receptors, sweat glands, oil glands	
24. Skeletal		Support, movement, storage of minerals, blood formation
25. Muscular	Muscles	
26.	Brain, spinal cord, nerves	Communication, integration, control, recognition of sensory stimuli
27. Endocrine		Secretion of hormones; communication, integration, control
28. Circulatory	Heart, blood vessels	
29. Lymphatic		Transportation, immunity
30.	Kidneys, ureters, bladder, urethra	Elimination of wastes, electrolyte balance, acid-base balance, water balance
31. Digestive		Digestion of food, absorption of nutrients
32.	Nose, pharynx, larynx, trachea, bronchi, lungs	Exchange of gases in the lungs, regulation of acid-base balance
33. Reproductive		Survival of species; production of sex cells, fertilization, development, birth; nourishment of offspring; production of hormones

If you have had difficulty with this section, review pages 79-92.

UNSCRAMBLE THE WORDS

Take the circled letters, unscramble them, and fill in the statement.

34. **RTAHE**

35. **IEPLNA**

36. **EENVR**

37. **SUHESOPGA**

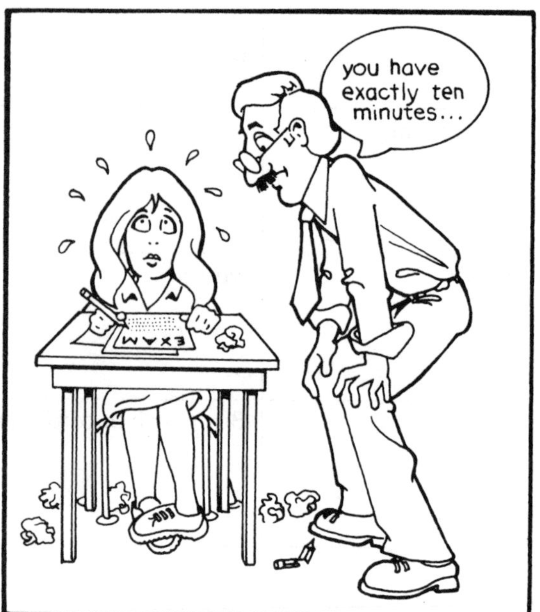

The more thoroughly you review this chapter, the less ________________ you will be during your test.

38.

APPLYING WHAT YOU KNOW

39. Myrna was 15 years old and had not yet started menstruating. Her family physician decided to consult two other physicians, each of whom specialized in a different system. Specialists in the areas of ____________________ and ____________________ were consulted.

40. Brian was admitted to the hospital with second- and third-degree burns that covered 50% of his body. He was placed in isolation, so when Jenny went to visit him, she was required to wear a hospital gown and mask. Why was Brian placed in isolation? Why was Jenny required to wear special attire?

41. WORD FIND

Can you find 11 organ systems? Words may be spelled top to bottom, bottom to top, right to left, left to right, or diagonally.

Y	R	A	T	N	E	M	U	G	E	T	N	I	R	F
H	N	E	R	V	O	U	S	K	I	R	J	M	G	T
L	Y	M	P	H	A	T	I	C	I	S	Y	Y	U	I
B	N	X	Y	R	O	T	A	L	U	C	R	I	C	W
P	E	L	R	E	O	M	J	M	S	O	M	M	P	S
C	C	W	M	A	N	D	L	A	T	E	L	E	K	S
R	R	K	E	M	L	I	U	A	A	V	V	U	K	N
D	K	X	P	D	J	U	R	C	J	I	R	Q	E	M
C	D	B	V	C	V	I	C	C	T	T	K	W	C	X
X	R	Q	Q	D	P	H	C	S	O	I	X	P	A	Z
M	F	M	U	S	Y	D	E	V	U	D	V	Y	K	E
U	E	S	E	C	Z	G	T	Q	D	M	N	E	K	O
P	Y	R	A	N	I	R	U	C	T	C	N	E	W	H
N	H	T	N	D	E	P	S	I	X	A	Q	O	I	E

Circulatory
Digestive
Endocrine
Integumentary
Lymphatic
Muscular
Nervous
Reproductive
Respiratory
Skeletal
Urinary

DID YOU KNOW?

Muscles comprise 40% of your body weight. Your skeleton, however, only accounts for 18% of your body weight.

Every person has a unique tongue print.

ORGAN SYSTEMS

Fill in the crossword puzzle.

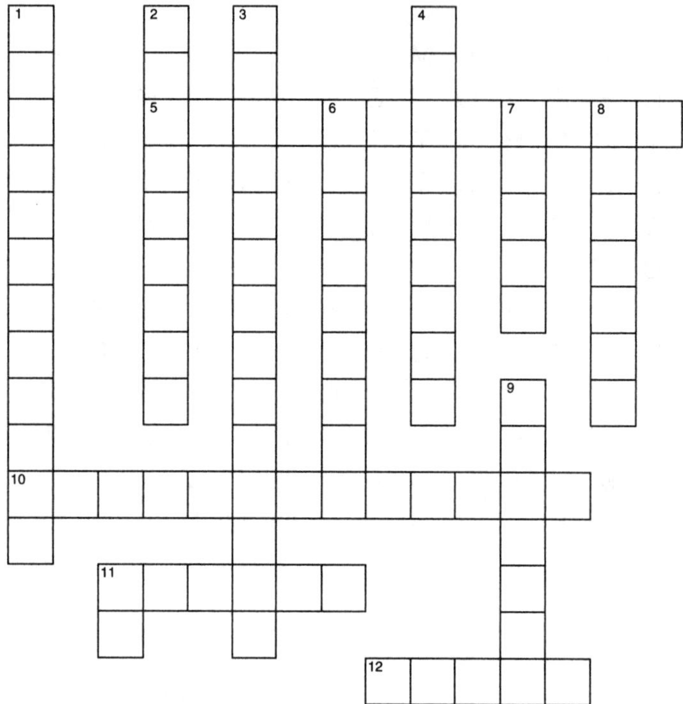

Across

5. Specialized signal of nervous system (two words)
10. Skin
11. Testes and ovaries
12. Undigested residue of digestion

Down

1. Inflammation of the appendix
2. Vulva, penis, and scrotum
3. Heart and blood vessels
4. Subdivision of circulatory system
6. System of hormones
7. Waste product of kidneys
8. Agent that causes change in the activity of a structure
9. Chemical secretion of endocrine system
11. Gastrointestinal tract (abbreviation)

CHECK YOUR KNOWLEDGE

Multiple Choice

Circle the correct answer.

1. Hormones belong to which body system?
   A. Nervous
   B. Integumentary
   C. Muscular
   D. Endocrine

2. The spleen belongs to which body system?
   A. Circulatory
   B. Urinary
   C. Lymphatic
   D. Digestive

3. Which of the following is *not* an accessory organ of the female reproductive system?
   A. Fallopian tubes
   B. Mammary glands
   C. Gonads
   D. Vagina

4. The largest and most complex structural units are:
   A. Cells
   B. Organs
   C. Tissues
   D. Nerve impulses

5. An important function of the skeletal system is:
   A. Recognition of sensory stimuli
   B. Regulation of acid-base balance in the body
   C. Elimination of wastes in the body
   D. Formation of blood cells

6. Appendages of the integumentary system include all of the following *except*:
   A. Hormones
   B. Sweat glands
   C. Oil-producing glands
   D. Nails

7. Which of the following is *not* a primary organ of the digestive system?
   A. Mouth
   B. Liver
   C. Esophagus
   D. Rectum

8. One of the primary functions of the nervous system is:
   A. Communication among body functions
   B. Protection
   C. Regulation of acid-base balance
   D. Secretion of hormones

9. Which of the following is *not* an endocrine gland?
   A. Vas deferens
   B. Thymus
   C. Pineal
   D. Pituitary

10. A structure made up of two or more kinds of tissues organized to perform a more complex function than any tissue alone is a(n):
    A. System
    B. Tissue
    C. Organ
    D. Cell

MATCHING

Select the most correct answer from column B for each statement in column A. (Only one answer is correct.)

Column A	Column B
_____ 11. Oil glands	A. Endocrine
_____ 12. Blood vessels	B. Urinary
_____ 13. Tonsils	C. Integumentary
_____ 14. Vas deferens	D. Circulatory
_____ 15. Ureters	E. Respiratory
_____ 16. Appendix	F. Digestive
_____ 17. Vulva	G. Male reproductive
_____ 18. Larynx	H. Lymphatic
_____ 19. Brain	I. Female reproductive
_____ 20. Thyroid	J. Nervous

SKELETAL SYSTEM

Fill in the crossword puzzle.

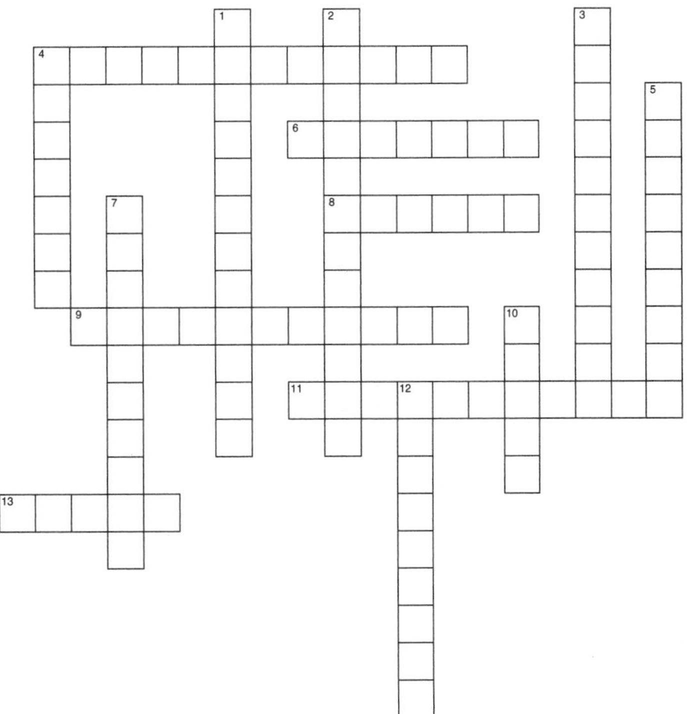

Across
4. Cartilage cells
6. Spaces in bones where osteocytes are found
8. Chest
9. Freely movable joints
11. Process of blood cell formation
13. Space inside cranial bone

Down
1. Joint
2. Suture joints
3. Bone absorbing cells
4. Type of bone
5. Ends of long bones
7. Covers long bone except at its joint surfaces
10. Division of skeleton
12. Bone cell

CHECK YOUR KNOWLEDGE

Multiple Choice

Circle the correct answer.

1. Which of the following is *not* a function of bones?
   A. Communication
   B. Storage
   C. Hemopoiesis
   D. Protection
2. The four types of bones are:
   A. Flat, irregular, short, and square
   B. Flat, cartilage, short, and long
   C. Flat, irregular, short, and long
   D. Small, long, flat, and heavy

3. Which of the following is *not* a main part of a long bone?
   A. Malleus
   B. Epiphyses
   C. Periosteum
   D. Diaphysis
4. All of the following bones are part of the appendicular skeleton *except*:
   A. Shoulder
   B. Hip
   C. Chest
   D. Feet
5. There are a total of _________ phalanges in the skeletal system.
   A. 28
   B. 60
   C. 56
   D. 72
6. Cartilage differs from bone because it:
   A. Is embedded in a firm gel rather than in a calcified cement substance
   B. Has the flexibility of a firm plastic rather than being rigid
   C. Rebuilds itself very slowly after injury
   D. All of the above
7. Which of the following is *not* a paranasal sinus?
   A. Frontal
   B. Ethmoid
   C. Lambdoidal
   D. Sphenoid
8. The last two ribs:
   A. Attach directly to the sternum
   B. Are attached to costal cartilage
   C. Are referred to as "floating ribs"
   D. None of the above
9. In an infant, each coxal bone consists of three separate bones. These bones are the:
   A. Ilium, ischium, and coccyx
   B. Ischium, pubis, and tuberosity
   C. Pubis, tuberosity, and coccyx
   D. Ilium, ischium, and pubis
10. An example of a synarthrotic joint is:
   A. A cranial suture
   B. The hip joint
   C. The shoulder joint
   D. The spine

Matching

Select the most correct answer from column B for each statement in column A. (Only one answer is correct.)

Column A	Column B
_____ 11. Articulation	A. "Funny bone"
_____ 12. Medullary cavity	B. Yellow bone marrow
_____ 13. Osteons	C. Immovable
_____ 14. Incus	D. Circumduct
_____ 15. Sternum	E. Manubrium
_____ 16. Zygomatic	F. Flexion
_____ 17. Olecranon process	G. Joint
_____ 18. Synarthroses	H. Cheekbone
_____ 19. Hinge joint	I. Haversian system
_____ 20. Thumb joint	J. Middle ear

POSTERIOR VIEW OF SKELETON

1. ______________________
2. ______________________
3. ______________________
4. ______________________
5. ______________________
6. ______________________
7. ______________________
8. ______________________
9. ______________________
10. ______________________
11. ______________________
12. ______________________
13. ______________________
14. ______________________

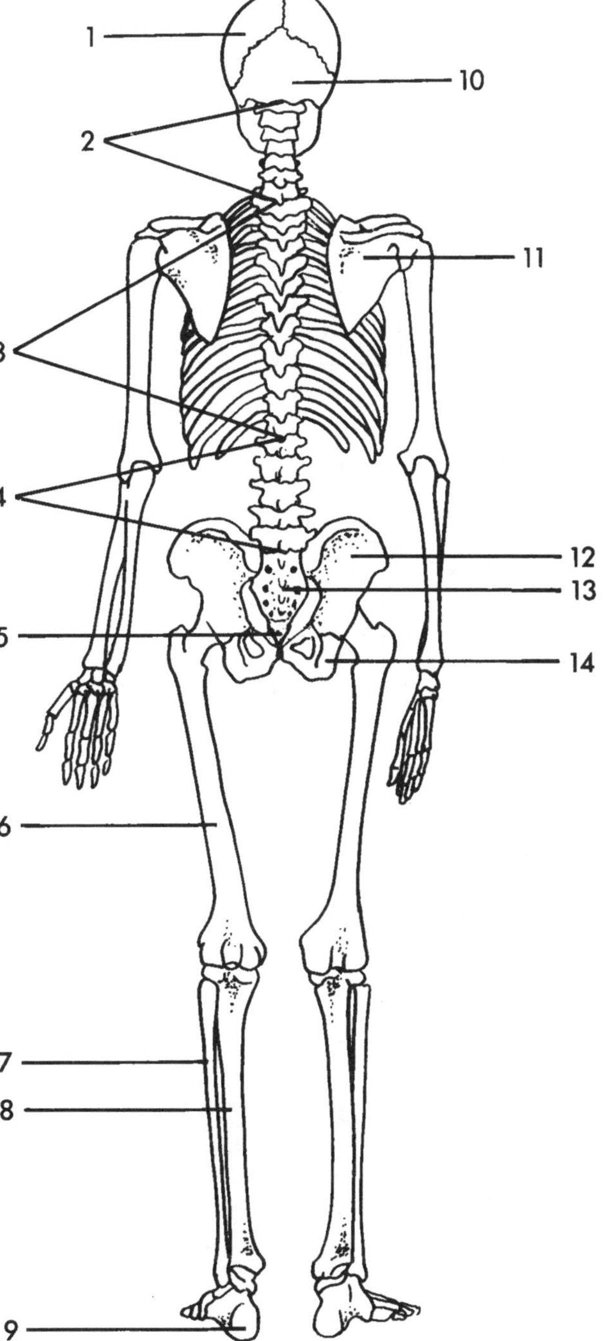

SKULL VIEWED FROM THE RIGHT SIDE

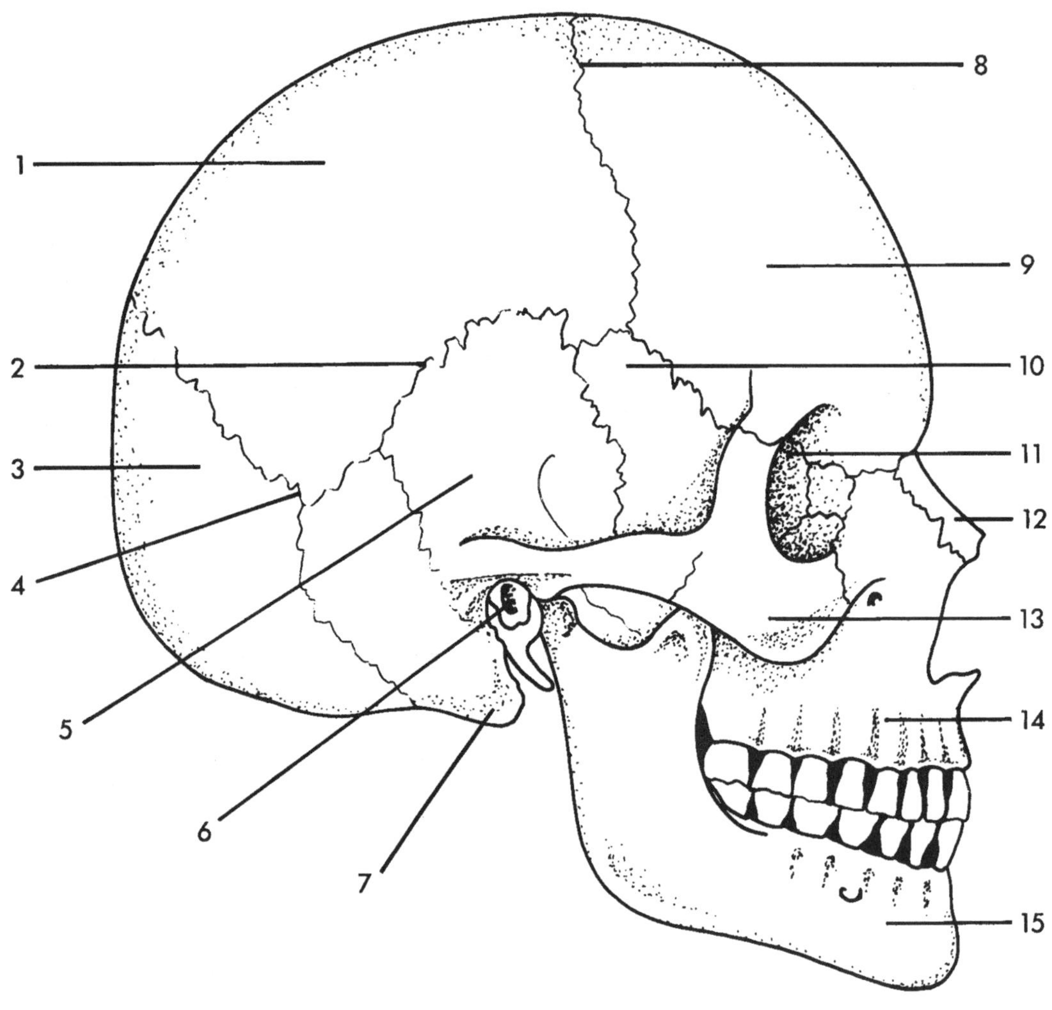

1. ______________________
2. ______________________
3. ______________________
4. ______________________
5. ______________________
6. ______________________
7. ______________________
8. ______________________
9. ______________________
10. ______________________
11. ______________________
12. ______________________
13. ______________________
14. ______________________
15. ______________________

SKULL VIEWED FROM THE FRONT

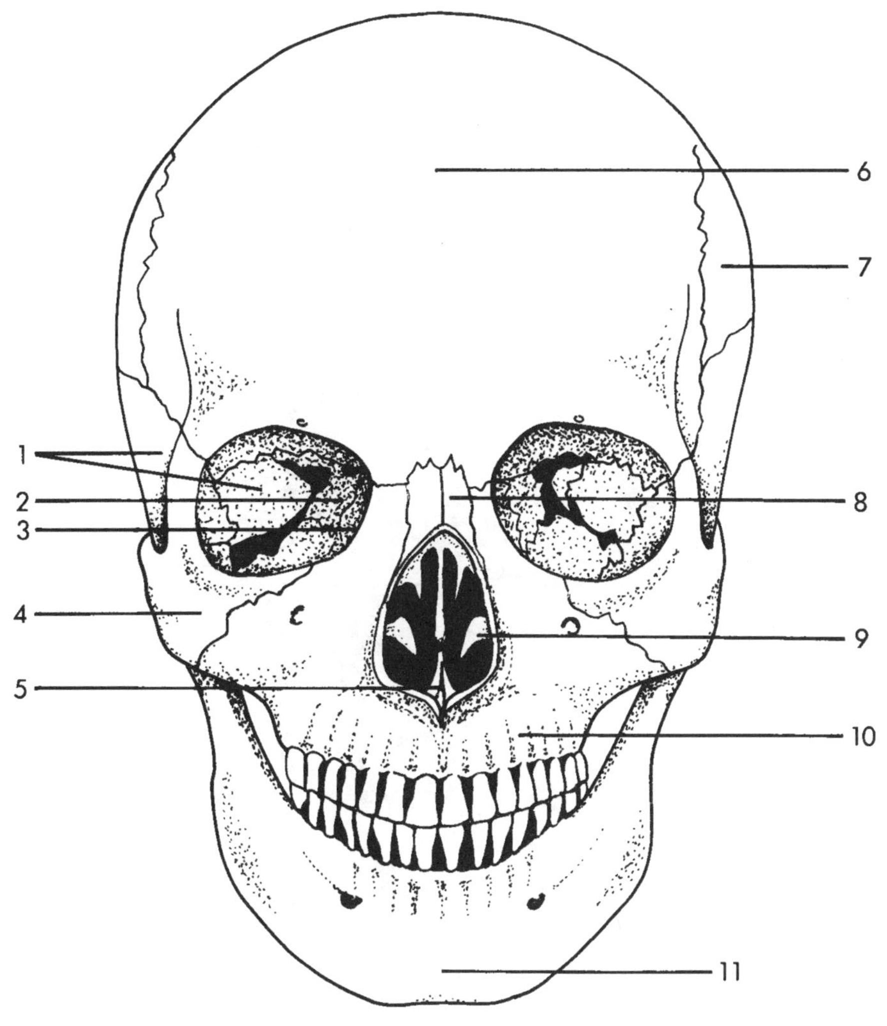

1. ______________________
2. ______________________
3. ______________________
4. ______________________
5. ______________________
6. ______________________
7. ______________________
8. ______________________
9. ______________________
10. ______________________
11. ______________________

STRUCTURE OF A DIARTHROTIC JOINT

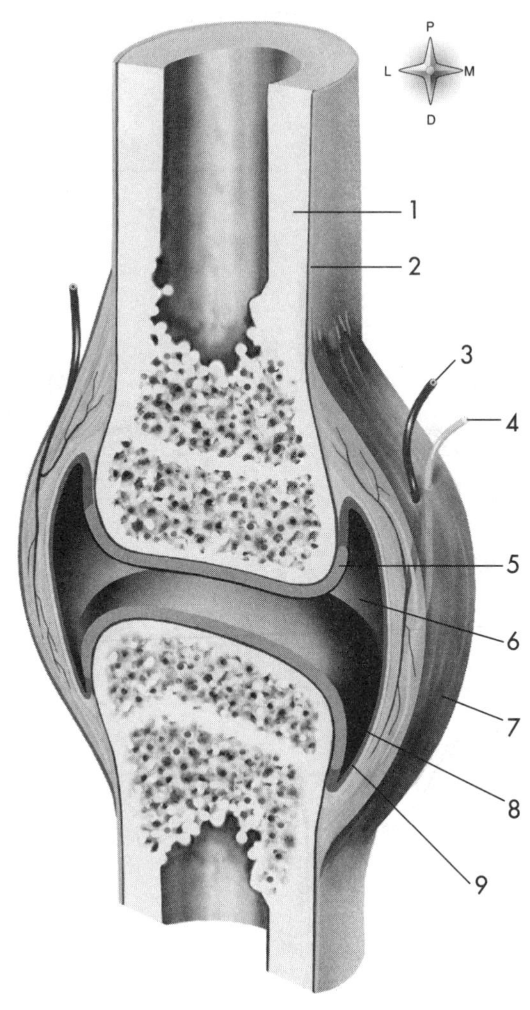

1. ______________________
2. ______________________
3. ______________________
4. ______________________
5. ______________________
6. ______________________
7. ______________________
8. ______________________
9. ______________________

THE MUSCULAR SYSTEM

Fill in the crossword puzzle.

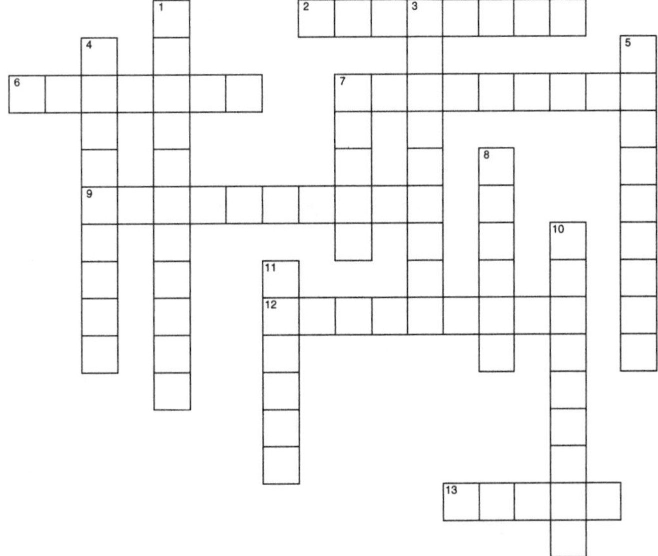

Across

2. Shaking your head "no"
6. Muscle shrinkage
7. Toward the body's midline
9. Produces movement opposite to prime movers
12. Movement that makes joint angles larger
13. Small fluid-filled sac between tendons and bones

Down

1. Increase in size
3. Away from the body's midline
4. Turning your palm from an anterior to posterior position
5. Attachment to the more movable bone
7. Protein that composes myofilaments
8. Attachment to the more stationary bone
10. Assists prime movers with movement
11. Anchors muscles to bones

CHECK YOUR KNOWLEDGE

Multiple Choice

Circle the correct answer.

1. Endurance training is also called:
   A. Isometrics
   B. Hypertrophy
   C. Anaerobic training
   D. Aerobic training
2. Increase in muscle size is called:
   A. Hypertrophy
   B. Atrophy
   C. Hyperplasia
   D. Treppe

3. Which of the following statements concerning isometric contractions is true?
   A. Walking is an example of an isometric contraction.
   B. Muscle tension decreases.
   C. Muscle length remains constant.
   D. Movement of the muscle increases.
4. Muscle cells are stimulated by a nerve fiber called a:
   A. Sarcomere
   B. Motor neuron
   C. Myofilament
   D. Prime mover
5. Muscles that help other muscles produce movement are called:
   A. Synergists
   B. Prime movers
   C. Antagonists
   D. None of the above
6. The connecting bridges between myofilaments form properly only if ________ is present.
   A. Potassium
   B. Calcium
   C. Sodium
   D. Chloride
7. Physiological muscle fatigue is caused by:
   A. Oxygen debt
   B. Lack of ATP
   C. Lactic acid buildup in the muscles
   D. All of the above
8. The muscle's attachment to the more stationary bone is called its:
   A. Origin
   B. Body
   C. Insertion
   D. None of the above
9. Skeletal muscle:
   A. Is voluntary
   B. Is smooth
   C. Is also known as visceral muscle
   D. All of the above
10. Which of the following is *not* a hamstring muscle?
   A. Semimembranosus
   B. Semitendinosus
   C. Rectus femoris
   D. Biceps femoris

True or False

Indicate whether the following statements are true (T) or false (F).

_____ 11. The "all or none" principle states that when a muscle fiber is subjected to a threshold stimulus, it contracts completely.
_____ 12. Muscle tone maintains posture.
_____ 13. Thick myofilaments are formed from a protein called actin.
_____ 14. The triceps brachii is on the anterior surface of the upper arm.
_____ 15. Tendons anchor muscles firmly to bones.
_____ 16. Energy required to produce a muscle contraction is obtained from ATP.
_____ 17. Rotation is movement around a longitudinal axis.
_____ 18. Extension movements are the opposite of abduction.
_____ 19. The gastrocnemius is responsible for plantar flexion of the foot and is sometimes referred to as the "toe dancer's muscle."
_____ 20. The zygomaticus is sometimes called the "kissing muscle."

MUSCLES—ANTERIOR VIEW

1. ______________________________
2. ______________________________
3. ______________________________
4. ______________________________
5. ______________________________

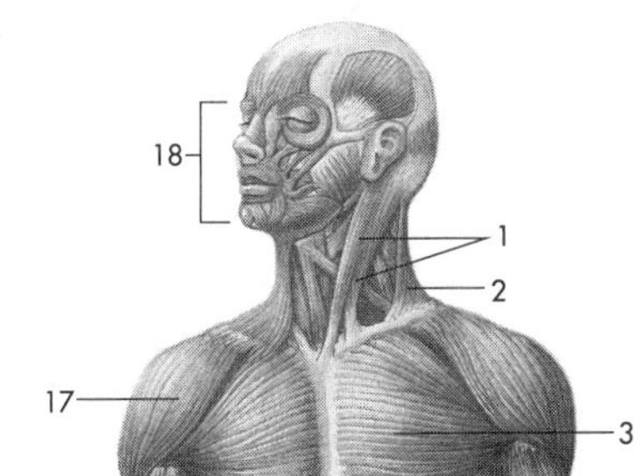

MUSCLES—POSTERIOR VIEW

1. ______________________________
2. ______________________________
3. ______________________________
4. ______________________________
5. ______________________________
6. ______________________________
7. ______________________________
8. ______________________________
9. ______________________________
10. ______________________________
11. ______________________________
12. ______________________________
13. ______________________________

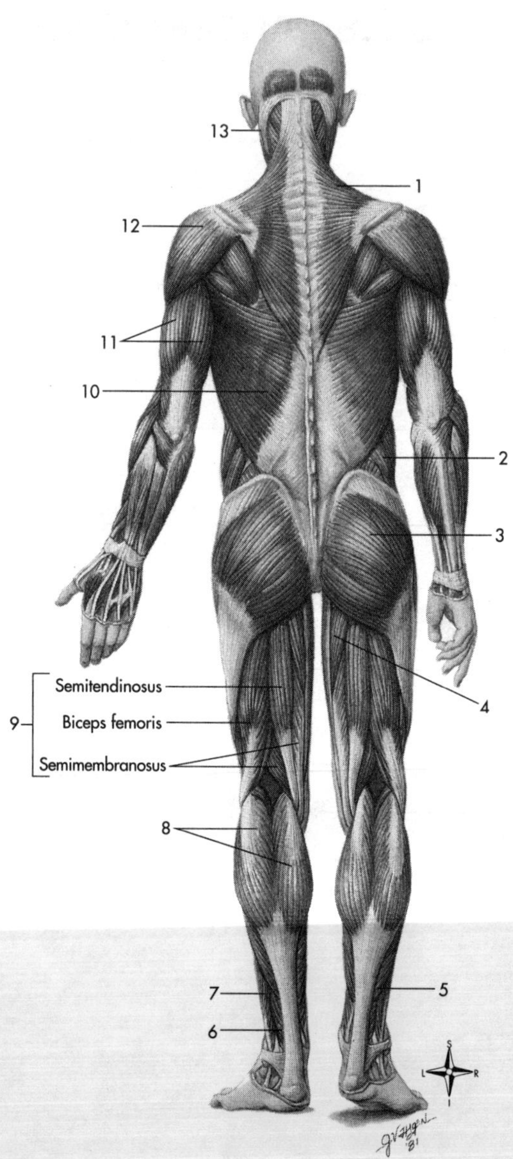

CHAPTER 8

The Nervous System

The nervous system organizes and coordinates the millions of impulses received each day to make communication with and enjoyment of our environment possible. The functioning unit of the nervous system is the neuron. Three types of neurons—sensory neurons, motor neurons, and interneurons—exist, and are classified according to the direction in which they transmit impulses. Nerve impulses travel over routes made up of neurons and provide the rapid communication necessary for maintaining life. The central nervous system is made up of the spinal cord and brain. The spinal cord provides access to and from the brain by means of ascending and descending tracts. In addition, the spinal cord functions as the primary reflex center of the body. The brain can be subdivided for easier learning into the brain stem, cerebellum, diencephalon, and cerebrum. These areas provide the extraordinary network necessary to receive, interpret, and respond to the simplest or most complex impulses.

While you concentrate on this chapter, your body is performing a multitude of functions. Fortunately for us, breathing, beating of the heart, digestion of food, and most of our other day-to-day processes do not require our supervision or thought. They function automatically, and the division of the nervous system that regulates these functions is known as the autonomic nervous system.

The autonomic nervous system consists of two divisions called the sympathetic system and the parasympathetic system. The sympathetic system functions as an emergency system and prepares us for "fight or flight." The parasympathetic system dominates control of many visceral effectors under normal everyday conditions. Together, these two divisions regulate the body's automatic functions in an effort to assist with the maintenance of homeostasis. Your understanding of this chapter will alert you to the complexity and functions of the nervous system and the "automatic pilot" of your body—the autonomic system.

TOPICS FOR REVIEW

Before progressing to Chapter 9, you should review the organs and divisions of the nervous system, the structure and function of the major types of cells in this system, the structure and function of a reflex arc, and the transmission of nerve impulses. Your study should include the anatomy and physiology of the brain and spinal cord and the nerves that extend from these two areas.

Finally, an understanding of the autonomic nervous system and the specific functions of the subdivisions of this system are necessary to complete the review of this chapter.

ORGANS AND DIVISIONS OF THE NERVOUS SYSTEM
CELLS OF THE NERVOUS SYSTEM
NERVES

Match the term on the left with the proper selection on the right.

Group A

Answer	Term		Selection
B	1. Sense organ	A.	Subdivision of peripheral nervous system
C	2. Central nervous system	B.	Ear
D	3. Peripheral nervous system	C.	Brain and spinal cord
A	4. Autonomic nervous system	D.	Nerves that extend to the outlying parts of the body

Group B

Answer	Term		Selection
B	5. Dendrite	A.	Indentations between adjacent Schwann cells
D	6. Schwann cell	B.	Branching projection of neuron
C	7. Motor neuron	C.	Also known as "efferent"
A	8. Nodes of Ranvier	D.	Forms myelin outside the central nervous system
F	9. Fascicles	E.	Tough sheath that covers the whole nerve
E	10. Epineurium	F.	Groups of wrapped axons

CELLS OF NERVOUS SYSTEM

Select the correct term from the choices given and write the letter in the answer blank.

(A) Neurons (B) Neuroglia

A 11. Axon

B 12. Special type of supporting cells

B 13. Astrocytes

A 14. Sensory

A 15. Conduct impulses

B 16. Forms the myelin sheath around central nerve fibers

B 17. Phagocytosis

A 18. Efferent

B 19. Multiple sclerosis

A 20. Neurilemma

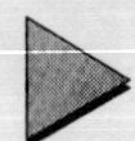
If you have had difficulty with this section, review pages 185-190.

REFLEX ARCS

Fill in the blanks.

21. The simplest kind of reflex arc is a ______________________.
22. Three-neuron arcs consist of all three kinds of neurons, __________, __________, and __________.
23. Impulse conduction in a reflex arc normally starts in __________.
24. A __________ is the microscopic space that separates the axon of one neuron from the dendrites of another neuron.
25. A __________ is the response to impulse conduction over reflex arcs.
26. Contraction of a muscle that causes it to pull away from an irritating stimulus is known as the __________.
27. A __________ is a group of nerve cell bodies located in the peripheral nervous system.
28. All __________ lie entirely within the gray matter of the central nervous system.
29. In a patellar reflex, the nerve impulses that reach the quadriceps muscle (the effector) result in the classic "__________" response.
30. __________ forms the H-shaped inner core of the spinal cord.

If you have had difficulty with this section, review pages 190-193.

NERVE IMPULSES THE SYNAPSE

Circle the correct answer.

31. Nerve impulses (do or do not) continually race along every nerve cell's surface.
32. When a stimulus acts on a neuron, it (increases or decreases) the permeability of the stimulated point of its membrane to sodium ions.
33. An inward movement of positive ions leaves (a lack or an excess) of negative ions outside.
34. The plasma membrane of the (presynaptic or postsynaptic) neuron makes up a portion of the synapse.
35. A synaptic knob is a tiny bulge at the end of the (presynaptic or postsynaptic) neuron's axon.
36. Acetylcholine is an example of a (neurotransmitter or protein molecule receptor).
37. Neurotransmitters are chemicals that allow neurons to (communicate or reproduce) with one another.
38. Neurotransmitters are distributed (randomly or specifically) into groups of neurons.
39. Catecholamines may play a role in (sleep or reproduction).
40. Endorphins and enkephalins are neurotransmitters that inhibit conduction of (fear or pain) impulses.

If you have had difficulty with this section, review pages 193-196.

CENTRAL NERVOUS SYSTEM
DIVISIONS OF THE BRAIN

Circle the correct answer.

41. The portion of the brain stem that joins the spinal cord to the brain is the:
    A. Pons
    B. Cerebellum
    C. Diencephalon
    D. Hypothalamus
    E. Medulla

42. Which one of the following is *not* a function of the brain stem?
    A. Conduction of sensory impulses from the spinal cord to the higher centers of the brain
    B. Conduction of motor impulses from the cerebrum to the spinal cord
    C. Control of heartbeat, respiration, and blood vessel diameter
    D. Containment of centers for speech and memory

43. Which one of the following is *not* part of the diencephalon?
    A. Cerebrum
    B. Thalamus
    C. Hypothalamus
    D. All of the above are correct

44. ADH is produced by the:
    A. Pituitary gland
    B. Medulla
    C. Mammillary bodies
    D. Third ventricle
    E. Hypothalamus

45. Which one of the following is *not* true about the hypothalamus?
    A. It helps control the rate of heartbeat.
    B. It helps control the constriction and dilation of blood vessels.
    C. It helps control the contraction of the stomach and intestines.
    D. It produces releasing hormones that control the release of certain anterior pituitary hormones.
    E. All of the above are true.

46. Which one of the following parts of the brain helps in the association of sensations with emotions and also aids in the arousal or alerting mechanism?
    A. Pons
    B. Hypothalamus
    C. Cerebellum
    D. Thalamus
    E. None of the above

47. Which of the following is *not* true of the cerebrum?
    A. Its lobes correspond to the bones that lie over them.
    B. Its grooves are called gyri.
    C. Most of its gray matter lies on the surface of the cerebrum.
    D. Its outer region is called the cerebral cortex.
    E. Its two hemispheres are connected by a structure called the corpus callosum.

48. Which one of the following is *not* a function of the cerebrum?
    A. Willed movement
    B. Consciousness
    C. Memory
    D. Conscious awareness of sensations
    E. All of the above are functions of the cerebrum

49. The area of the cerebrum responsible for the perception of sound lies in the ________________ lobe.
    A. Frontal
    B. Temporal
    C. Occipital
    D. Parietal

50. Visual perception is located in the ______________________ lobe.
    A. Frontal
    B. Temporal
    C. Parietal
    D. Occipital
    E. None of the above

51. Which one of the following is *not* a function of the cerebellum?
    A. Maintains equilibrium
    B. Helps with production of smooth, coordinated movements
    C. Helps maintain normal postures
    D. Associates sensations with emotions

52. Within the interior of the cerebrum are a few islands of gray matter known as:
    A. Fissures
    B. Basal ganglia
    C. Gyri
    D. Myelin

53. A cerebrovascular accident is commonly referred to as:
    A. A stroke
    B. Parkinson's disease
    C. A tumor
    D. Multiple sclerosis

54. Parkinson's disease is a disease of the:
    A. Myelin
    B. Axons
    C. Neuroglia
    D. Cerebral nuclei

55. The largest section of the brain is the:
    A. Cerebellum
    B. Pons
    C. Cerebrum
    D. Midbrain

If you have had difficulty with this section, review pages 196-202.

SPINAL CORD

If the statement is true, write "T" in the answer blank. If the statement is false, correct the statement by circling the incorrect term and writing the correct term in the answer blank.

__________________ 56. The spinal cord is approximately 24–25 inches long.

__________________ 57. The spinal cord ends at the bottom of the sacrum.

__________________ 58. The extension of the meninges beyond the cord is convenient for performing CAT scans without danger of injuring the spinal cord.

__________________ 59. Bundles of myelinated nerve fibers (dendrites) make up the white outer columns of the spinal cord.

__________________ 60. Ascending tracts conduct impulses up the cord to the brain and descending tracts conduct impulses down the cord from the brain.

__________________ 61. Tracts are functional organizations in that all the axons that compose a tract serve several functions.

__________________ 62. A loss of sensation caused by a spinal cord injury is called paralysis.

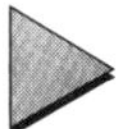
If you have had difficulty with this section, review pages 202-205.

COVERINGS AND FLUID SPACES OF BRAIN AND SPINAL CORD

Circle the one that does not *belong.*

63. Meninges	Pia mater	Ventricles	Dura mater
64. Arachnoid	Middle layer	CSF	Cobweb-like
65. CSF	Ventricles	Subarachnoid space	Pia mater
66. Tough	Outer layer	Dura mater	Choroid plexus
67. Brain tumor	Subarachnoid space	CSF	Fourth lumbar vertebra

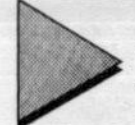
If you have had difficulty with this section, review pages 205-208.

PERIPHERAL NERVOUS SYSTEM—CRANIAL NERVES

68. *Fill in the missing areas on the chart below.*

NERVE		CONDUCT IMPULSES	FUNCTION
I		From nose to brain	Sense of smell
II	Optic		From eye to brain
III	Oculomotor		Eye movements
IV		From brain to external eye muscles	Eye movements
V	Trigeminal	From skin and mucous membrane of head and from teeth to brain; also from brain to chewing muscles	
VI	Abducens		Eye movements
VII	Facial	From taste buds of tongue to brain; from brain to face muscles	
VIII		From ear to brain	Hearing; sense of balance
IX	Glossopharyngeal		Sensations of throat, taste, swallowing movements, secretion of saliva
X		From throat, larynx, and organs in thoracic and abdominal cavities to brain; also from brain to muscles of throat and to organs in thoracic and abdominal cavities	Sensations of throat, larynx, and of thoracic and abdominal organs; swallowing, voice production, slowing of heartbeat, acceleration of peristalsis (gut movements)
XI	Accessory	From brain to certain shoulder and neck muscles	
XII		From brain to muscles of tongue	Tongue movements

If you have had difficulty with this section, review page 210, Table 8-2.

CRANIAL NERVES
SPINAL NERVES

Select the correct term from the choices given and write its letter in the answer blank.

(A) Cranial nerves (B) Spinal nerves

_____ 69. 12 pairs

_____ 70. Dermatome

_____ 71. Vagus

_____ 72. Shingles

_____ 73. 31 pairs

_____ 74. Optic

_____ 75. C1

_____ 76. Plexus

If you have had difficulty with this section, review pages 208-210 and 216.

AUTONOMIC NERVOUS SYSTEM

Match the term on the left with the proper selection on the right.

_____	77. Autonomic nervous system	A.	Division of ANS
_____	78. Autonomic neurons	B.	Tissues to which autonomic neurons conduct impulses
_____	79. Preganglionic neurons	C.	Voluntary actions
_____	80. Visceral effectors	D.	Regulates body's involuntary functions
_____	81. Sympathetic system	E.	Motor neurons that make up the ANS
_____	82. Somatic nervous system	F.	Conduct impulses between the spinal cord and a ganglion

SYMPATHETIC NERVOUS SYSTEM
PARASYMPATHETIC NERVOUS SYSTEM

Circle the correct answer.

83. Dendrites and cell bodies of sympathetic preganglionic neurons are located in the:
   A. Brain stem and sacral portion of the spinal cord
   B. Sympathetic ganglia
   C. Gray matter of the thoracic and upper lumbar segments of the spinal cord
   D. Ganglia close to effectors

84. Which of the following statements is *not* correct?
   A. Sympathetic preganglionic neurons have their cell bodies located in the lateral gray column of certain parts of the spinal cord.
   B. Sympathetic preganglionic axons pass along the dorsal root of certain spinal nerves.
   C. There are synapses within sympathetic ganglia.
   D. Sympathetic responses are usually widespread, involving many organs.

85. Another name for the parasympathetic nervous system is:
    A. Thoracolumbar
    B. Craniosacral
    C. Visceral
    D. ANS
    E. Cholinergic

86. Which of the following statements is *not* correct?
    A. Sympathetic postganglionic neurons have their dendrites and cell bodies in sympathetic ganglia or collateral ganglia.
    B. Sympathetic ganglions are located in front of and at each side of the spinal column.
    C. Separate autonomic nerves distribute many sympathetic postganglionic axons to various internal organs.
    D. Very few sympathetic preganglionic axons synapse with postganglionic neurons.

87. Sympathetic stimulation usually results in:
    A. Response by numerous organs
    B. Response by only one organ
    C. Increased peristalsis
    D. Constriction of pupils

88. Parasympathetic stimulation frequently results in:
    A. Response by only one organ
    B. Responses by numerous organs
    C. The "fight or flight" response
    D. Increased heartbeat

Select the correct term from the choices given and write the letter in the answer blank.

(A) Sympathetic control (B) Parasympathetic control

_____ 89. Constricts pupils

_____ 90. Produces "goose pimples"

_____ 91. Increases sweat secretion

_____ 92. Increases secretion of digestive juices

_____ 93. Constricts blood vessels

_____ 94. Slows heartbeat

_____ 95. Relaxes bladder

_____ 96. Increases epinephrine secretion

_____ 97. Increases peristalsis

_____ 98. Stimulates lens for near vision

If you have had difficulty with this section, review pages 210-215.

AUTONOMIC NEUROTRANSMITTERS
AUTONOMIC NERVOUS SYSTEM AS A WHOLE

Fill in the blanks.

99. Sympathetic preganglionic axons release the neurotransmitter ____________________.
100. Axons that release norepinephrine are classified as ______________ ______________.
101. Axons that release acetylcholine are classified as ______________ ______________.
102. The function of the autonomic nervous system is to regulate the body's involuntary functions in ways that maintain or restore ______________.
103. Your ______________ ____________________ is determined by the combined forces of the sympathetic and parasympathetic nervous system.
104. According to some physiologists, meditation leads to ____________________ sympathetic activity and changes opposite to those of the "fight or flight" response.

If you have had difficulty with this section, review pages 215-217.

UNSCRAMBLE THE WORDS

Take the circled letters, unscramble them, and fill in the statement.

105. **RONNESU**

106. **APSYENS**

107. **CIATUNOMO**

108. **SHTOMO ULMSEC**

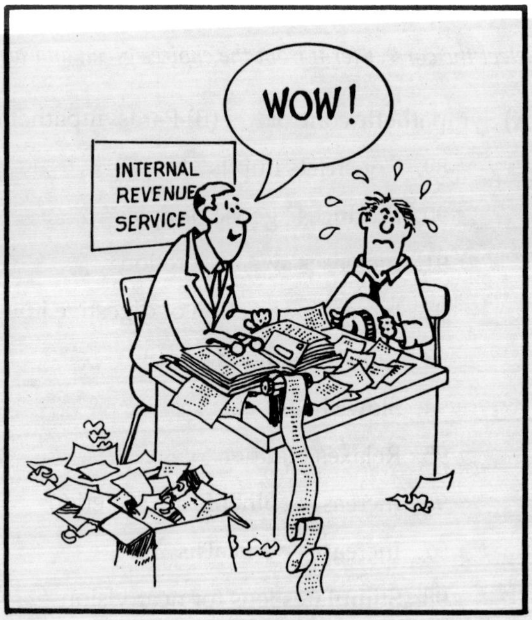

What the man hoped the IRS agent would be during his audit.

109.

APPLYING WHAT YOU KNOW

110. Mr. Hemstreet suffered a cerebrovascular accident and it was determined that the damage affected the left side of his cerebrum. On which side of his body will he most likely notice any paralysis?

111. Baby Dania was born with an excessive accumulation of cerebrospinal fluid in the ventricles. A catheter was placed in the ventricle and the fluid was drained by means of a shunt into the circulatory bloodstream. What condition does this medical history describe?

112. Mrs. Muhlenkamp looked out her window to see a man trapped under the wheel of a car. Although slightly built, Mrs. Muhlenkamp rushed to the car, lifted it, and saved the man underneath the wheel. What division of the autonomic nervous system made this seemingly impossible task possible?

113. Madison's heart raced and her palms became clammy as she watched the monster movie at the local theater. When the movie was over, however, she told her friends that she was not afraid at all. She appeared to be as calm as before the movie. What division of the autonomic nervous system made this possible?

114. Bill is going to his boss for his annual evaluation. He is planning to ask for a raise and hopes the evaluation will be good. Which subdivision of the autonomic nervous system will be active during this conference? Should he have a large meal before his appointment? Support your answer with facts from the chapter.

115. WORD FIND

Can you find the 14 terms from this chapter in the box of letters? Words may be spelled top to bottom, bottom to top, right to left, left to right, or diagonally.

M C C D Q S Y N A P S E Q G O

E N A Q D W H N W E J N A L W

S R O T P E C E R Y Z N I S M

I D S X E K N O K X G G C Y Y

J O T R A C T D F L O N E N A

R P W E K O H X I D A L H A M

F A L O N A Y O E I I I X P C

C M Z I F D N N L N G Z U T Z

S I N V C G D G Z A N A K I P

G N A T Z R O W V A M Y T C O

K E N D O R P H I N S I L C X

C P Q G C J X F J D Q S N L F

X U L I H I G Q A N S W O E U

A I M H Q E X K D B W Y T F S

A A D A X O C K G B F H B T K

Axon
Catecholamines
Dopamine
Endorphins
Ganglion
Glia
Microglia
Myelin
Oligodendroglia
Receptors
Serotonin
Synapse
Synaptic cleft
Tract

DID YOU KNOW?

Although all pain is felt and interpreted in the brain, it has no pain sensation itself—even when cut!

In the adult human body, there are 46 miles of nerves.

The areas of the brain that track emotion and memory are larger and more sensitive in the female brain.

"Rejection" actually hurts like physical pain because it triggers the same circuits in the brain.

THE NERVOUS SYSTEM

Fill in the crossword puzzle.

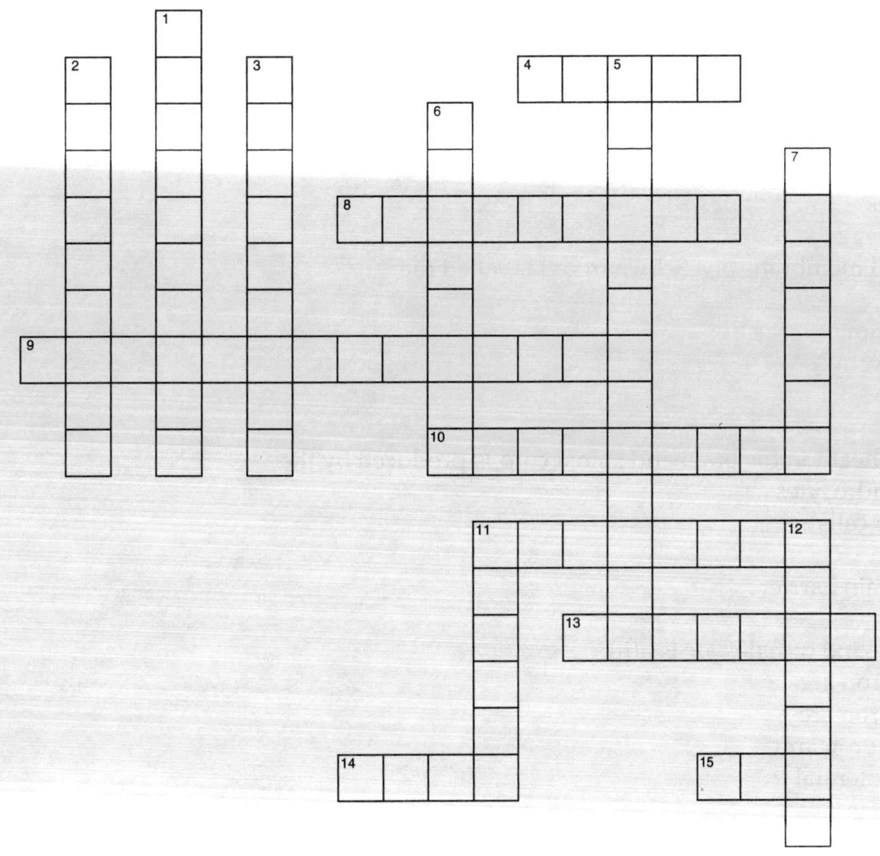

Across

4. Bundle of axons located within the CNS
8. Transmits impulses toward the cell body
9. Neurons that conduct impulses from a ganglion
10. Astrocytes
11. Pia mater
13. Nerve cells
14. Transmits impulses away from the cell body
15. Peripheral nervous system (abbreviation)

Down

1. Neuroglia
2. Peripheral beginning of a sensory neuron's dendrite
3. Two neuron arc (two words)
5. Neurotransmitter
6. Cluster of nerve cell bodies outside the central nervous system
7. Area of brain stem
11. Fatty substance found around some nerve fibers
12. Where impulses are transmitted from one neuron to another

CHECK YOUR KNOWLEDGE

Multiple Choice

Circle the correct answer.

1. Which of the following conducts impulses toward the cell body?
   A. Axons
   B. Astrocytes
   C. Microglia
   D. Dendrites

2. The outer cell membrane of a Schwann cell is called the:
   A. Glioma
   B. Neurilemma
   C. Cell body
   D. Dendrite

3. The myelin sheath in the brain and spinal cord is produced by the:
   A. Oligodendrocytes
   B. Schwann cells
   C. Microglia
   D. Blood-brain barrier

4. The simplest kind of reflex arc is a(n):
   A. One-neuron arc
   B. Two-neuron arc
   C. Three-neuron arc
   D. Action potential

5. A ganglion is a group of nerve cell bodies located in the:
   A. PNS
   B. CNS
   C. Brain and spinal cord
   D. All of the above

6. Each synaptic knob vesicle contains a very small quantity of a chemical compound called a:
   A. Synapse
   B. ADH
   C. Releasing hormone
   D. Neurotransmitter

7. Which of the following is located in the brain stem?
   A. Medulla oblongata
   B. Pons
   C. Midbrain
   D. All of the above

8. Which of the following is a function of the hypothalamus?
   A. Muscle coordination
   B. Willed movements
   C. Regulation of body temperature
   D. Relay for visual impulses

9. Which of the following is *not* true regarding the meninges?
   A. The tough outer layer is the dura mater.
   B. The arachnoid mater is the membrane between the dura mater and the pia mater.
   C. The pia mater resembles a "cobweb" and the name comes from the Greek word for spider.
   D. All of the above statements are true.

10. The autonomic nervous system consists of certain motor neurons that conduct impulses from the spinal cord or brain stem to the:
    A. Cardiac muscle tissue
    B. Smooth muscle tissue
    C. Glandular epithelial tissue
    D. All of the above

Matching

Select the most correct answer from column B for each statement in column A. (Only one answer is correct.)

Column A	Column B
_____ 11. Multiple sclerosis	A. Corpus callosum
_____ 12. Cerebrum	B. Abducens
_____ 13. CVA	C. Myelin disorder
_____ 14. Cerebrospinal fluid	D. Slows heartbeat
_____ 15. Cranial nerves	E. "Fight or flight"
_____ 16. Spinal nerves	F. Visceral effectors
_____ 17. Autonomic neurons	G. Parkinson's disease
_____ 18. Sympathetic nervous system	H. Ventricles
_____ 19. Parasympathetic nervous system	I. Thirty-one pairs
_____ 20. Dopamine	J. Stroke

NEURON

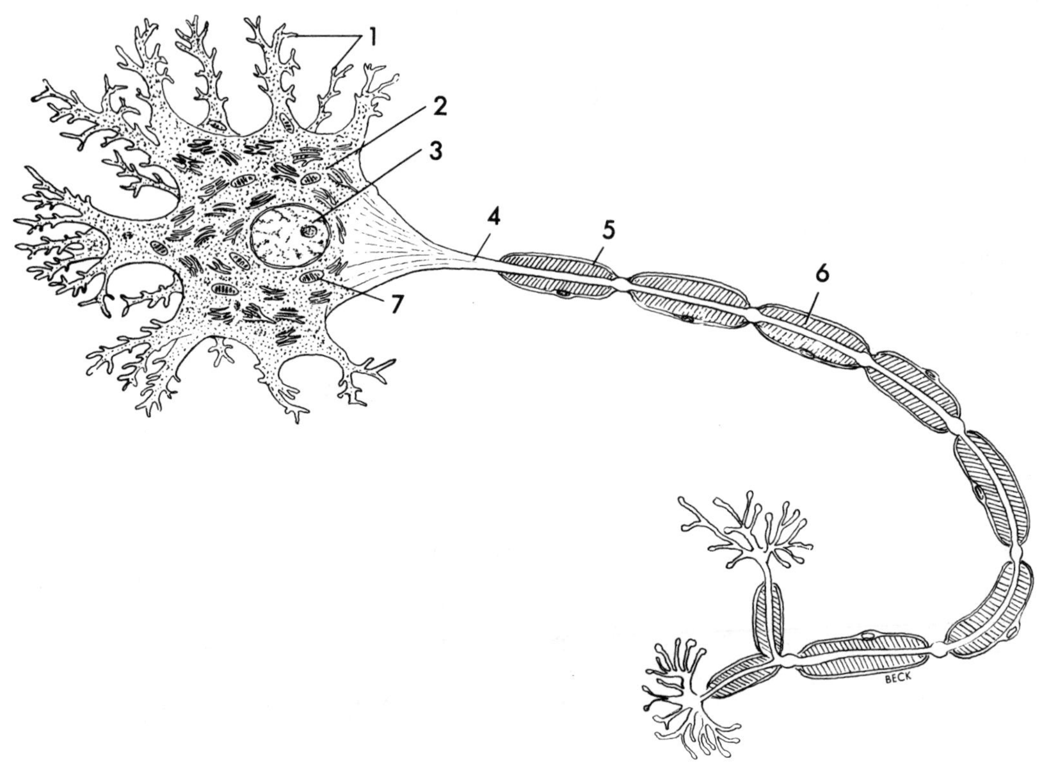

1. ______________________
2. ______________________
3. ______________________
4. ______________________
5. ______________________
6. ______________________
7. ______________________

CRANIAL NERVES

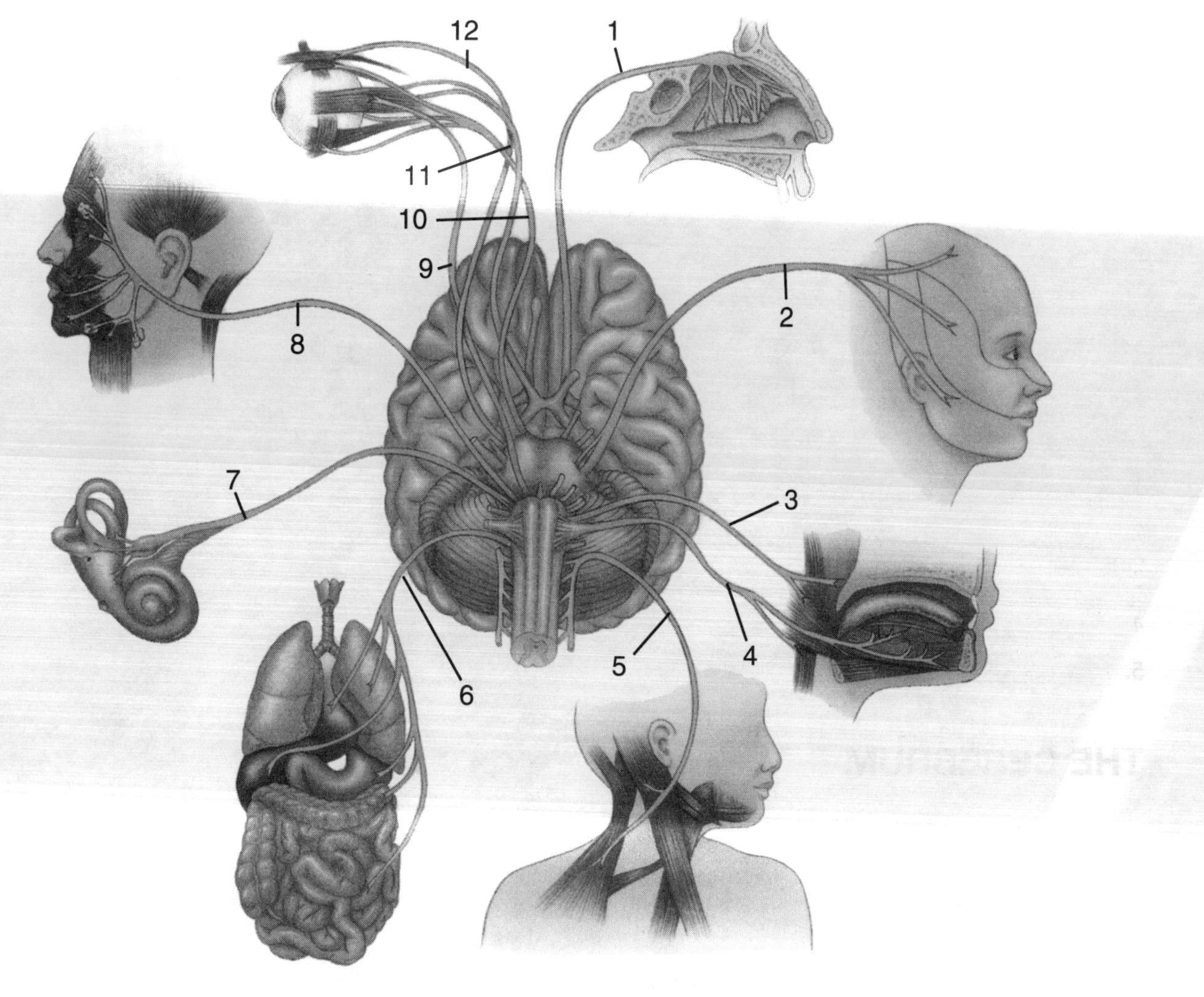

1. ______________________
2. ______________________
3. ______________________
4. ______________________
5. ______________________
6. ______________________
7. ______________________
8. ______________________
9. ______________________
10. ______________________
11. ______________________
12. ______________________

NEURAL PATHWAY INVOLVED IN THE PATELLAR REFLEX

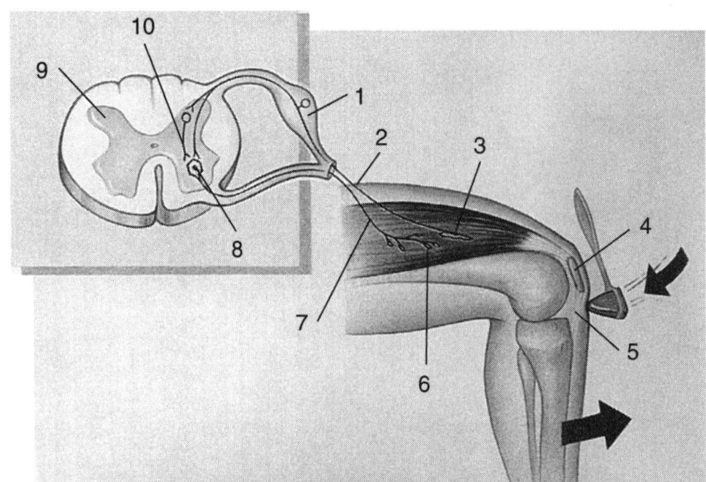

1. ____________________ 6. ____________________

2. ____________________ 7. ____________________

3. ____________________ 8. ____________________

4. ____________________ 9. ____________________

____________________ 10. ____________________

E CEREBRUM

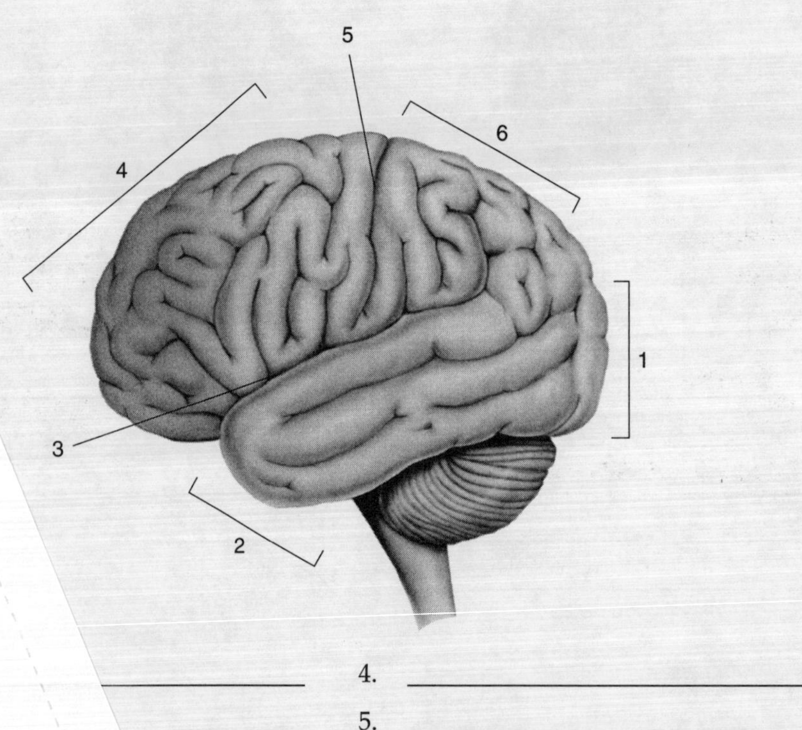

1. ____________________ 4. ____________________

2. ____________________ 5. ____________________

3. ____________________ 6. ____________________

SAGITTAL SECTION OF THE CENTRAL NERVOUS SYSTEM

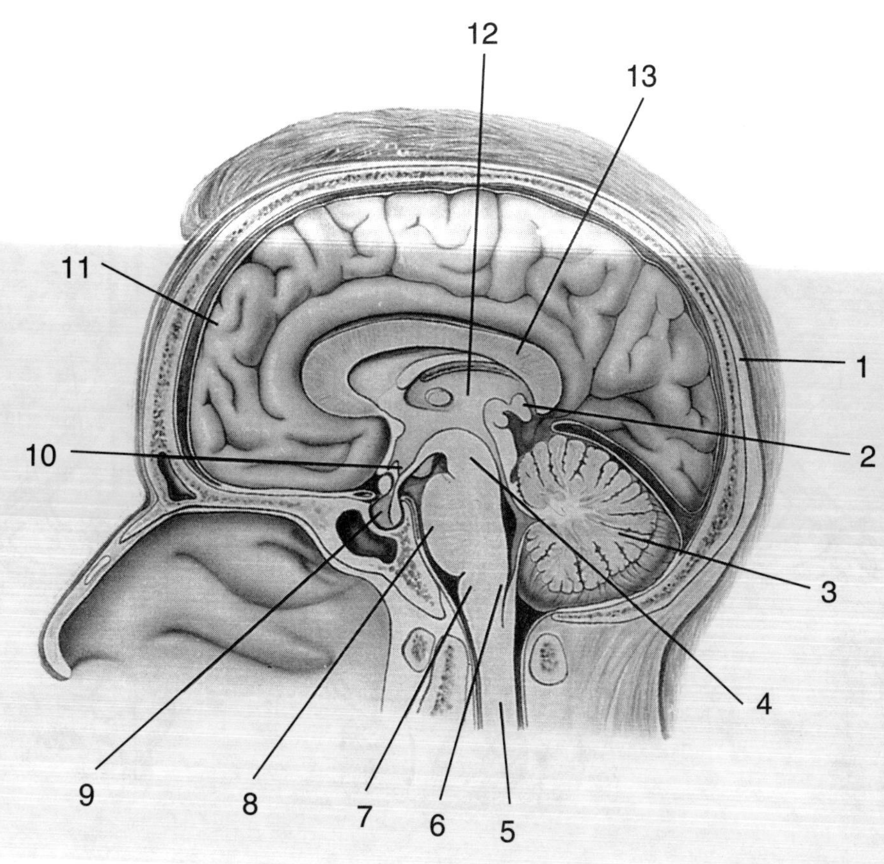

1. Skull
2. pineal gland
3. cerebum
4. mid brain
5. spinal cord
6. medulla
7. rectioular formation
8. pons
9. pituitary gland
10. hypothalmus
11. cerebral cortex
12. thalmus
13. corpus callsum

AUTONOMIC CONDUCTION PATHS

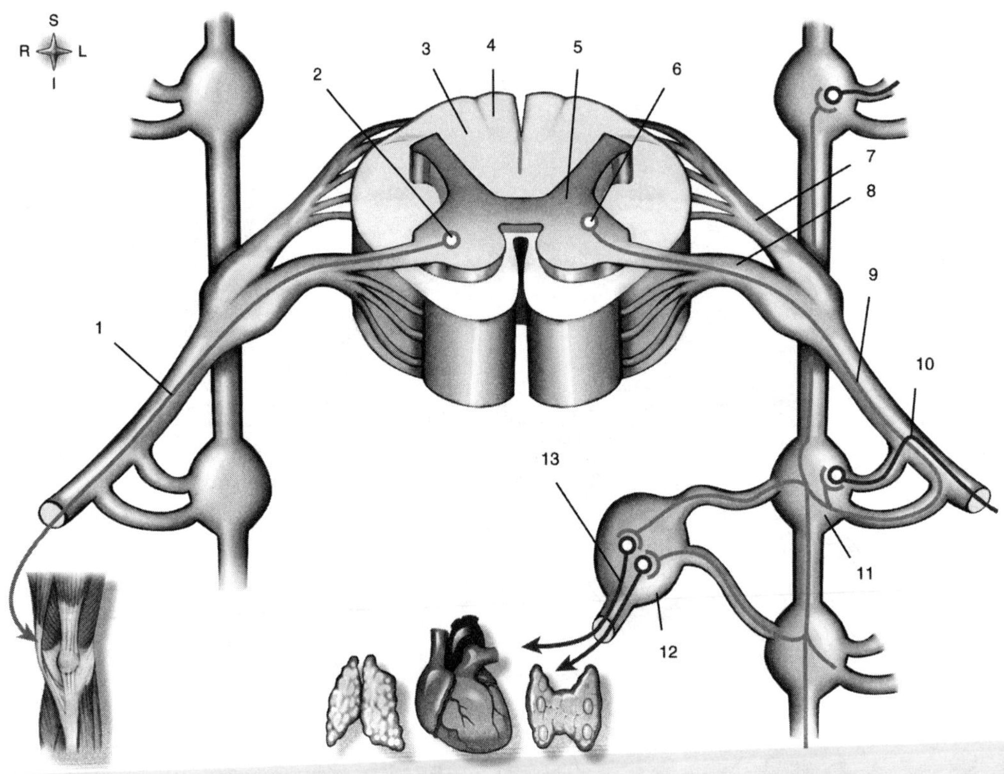

1. ______________________
2. ______________________
3. ______________________
4. ______________________
5. ______________________
6. ______________________
7. ______________________
8. ______________________
9. ______________________
10. ______________________
11. ______________________
12. ______________________
13. ______________________

CHAPTER 9

The Senses

Consider this scene for a moment. You are walking along a beautiful beach watching the sunset. You notice the various hues and are amazed at the multitude of shades that cover the sky. The waves are indeed melodious as they splash along the shore, and you wiggle your feet with delight as you sense the warm, soft sand trickling between your toes. You sip on a soda and then inhale the fresh salt air as you continue your stroll along the shore. It is a memorable scene, but one that would not be possible without the assistance of your sense organs. The sense organs pick up messages that are sent over nerve pathways to specialized areas in the brain for interpretation. They make communication with and enjoyment of the environment possible. The visual, auditory, tactile, olfactory, and gustatory sense organs not only protect us from danger but also add an important dimension to our daily pleasures of life.

Your study of this chapter will give you an understanding of another of the systems necessary for homeostasis and survival.

TOPICS FOR REVIEW

Before progressing to Chapter 10, you should review the classification of sense organs and the process for converting a stimulus into a sensation. Your study should also include an understanding of the special sense organs and the general sense organs.

CLASSIFICATION OF SENSE ORGANS
CONVERTING A STIMULUS INTO A SENSATION
GENERAL SENSE ORGANS

Match the term on the left with the proper selection on the right.

D 1. Special sense organ — A. Olfactory cells

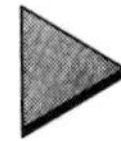

B 2. General sense organ — B. Meissner's corpuscles

A 3. Nose — C. Chemoreceptor

E 4. Krause's end-bulbs — D. Eye

C 5. Taste buds — E. Touch

If you have had difficulty with this section, review pages 227-231.

SPECIAL SENSE ORGANS

Eye

Circle the correct answer.

6. The "white" of the eye is more commonly called the:
   A. Choroid
   B. Cornea
   C. Sclera
   D. Retina
   E. None of the above

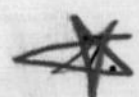

7. The "colored" part of the eye is known as the:
   A. Retina
   B. Cornea
   C. Pupil
   D. Sclera
   E. Iris

8. The transparent portion of the sclera, referred to as the "window" of the eye, is the:
   A. Retina
   B. Cornea
   C. Pupil
   D. Iris

9. The mucous membrane that covers the front of the eye is called the:
   A. Cornea
   B. Choroid
   C. Conjunctiva
   D. Ciliary body
   E. None of the above

10. The structure that can contract or dilate to allow more or less light to enter the eye is the:
    A. Lens
    B. Choroid
    C. Retina
    D. Cornea
    E. Iris

11. When the eye is looking at objects far in the distance, the lens is __________________ and the ciliary muscle is __________________.
    A. Rounded; contracted
    B. Rounded; relaxed
    C. Slightly rounded; contracted
    D. Slightly curved; relaxed
    E. None of the above

12. The lens of the eye is held in place by the:
    A. Ciliary muscle
    B. Aqueous humor
    C. Vitreous humor
    D. Cornea

13. When the lens loses its elasticity and can no longer bring near objects into focus, the condition is known as:
    A. Glaucoma
    B. Presbyopia
    C. Astigmatism
    D. Strabismus

14. The fluid in front of the lens that is constantly being formed, drained, and replaced in the anterior chamber is the:
    A. Vitreous humor
    B. Protoplasm
    C. Aqueous humor
    D. Conjunctiva

15. If drainage of the aqueous humor is blocked, the internal pressure within the eye will increase and a condition known as __________________ could occur.
    A. Presbyopia
    B. Glaucoma
    C. Color blindness
    D. Cataracts

16. The rods and cones are the photoreceptor cells and are located on the:
    A. Sclera
    B. Cornea
    C. Choroid
    D. Retina

17. The area which contains the greatest concentration of cones on the retina is the:
    A. Fovea centralis
    B. Retinal artery
    C. Ciliary body
    D. Optic disc

18. If our eyes are abnormally elongated, the image focuses in front of the retina and a condition known as __________________ occurs.
    A. Hyperopia
    B. Cataracts
    C. Night blindness
    D. Myopia

If you have had difficulty with this section, review pages 231-236.

Ear

Select the correct term from the choices given and write the letter in the answer blank.

(A) External ear (B) Middle ear (C) Inner ear

_____ 19. Malleus
_____ 20. Perilymph
_____ 21. Incus
_____ 22. Ceruminous glands
_____ 23. Cochlea
_____ 24. Auditory canal
_____ 25. Semicircular canals
_____ 26. Stapes
_____ 27. Eustachian tube
_____ 28. Organ of Corti

Fill in the blanks.

29. The external ear has two parts: the __________ and the __________ __________.
30. Another name for the tympanic membrane is the __________.
31. The bones of the middle ear are collectively referred to as __________.
32. The stapes presses against a membrane that covers a small opening called the __________ __________.
33. A middle ear infection is called __________ __________.
34. The __________ is located adjacent to the oval window between the semicircular canals and the cochlea.
35. Located within the semicircular canals and the vestibule are __________ for balance and equilibrium.
36. The sensory cells in the __________ __________ are stimulated when movement of the head causes the endolymph to move.

If you have had difficulty with this section, review pages 236-241.

TASTE RECEPTORS SMELL RECEPTORS

Circle the correct answer.

37. Structures known as (papillae or olfactory cells) are found on the tongue.
38. Nerve impulses generated by stimulation of taste buds travel primarily through two (cranial or spinal) nerves.
39. To be detected by olfactory receptors, chemicals must be dissolved in the watery (mucus or plasma) that lines the nasal cavity.
40. The pathways taken by olfactory nerve impulses and the areas where these impulses are interpreted are closely associated with areas of the brain important in (hearing or memory).
41. (Chemoreceptor or mechanoreceptor) is the term used to describe the type of receptors that generate nervous impulses resulting in the sense of taste or smell.

If you have had difficulty with this section, review pages 241-245.

UNSCRAMBLE THE WORDS

Take the circled letters, unscramble them, and fill in the statement.

42. **C A L R I E U**

43. **R A E C L S**

44. **L A P I L A E P**

45. **C T V N U C N O I A J**

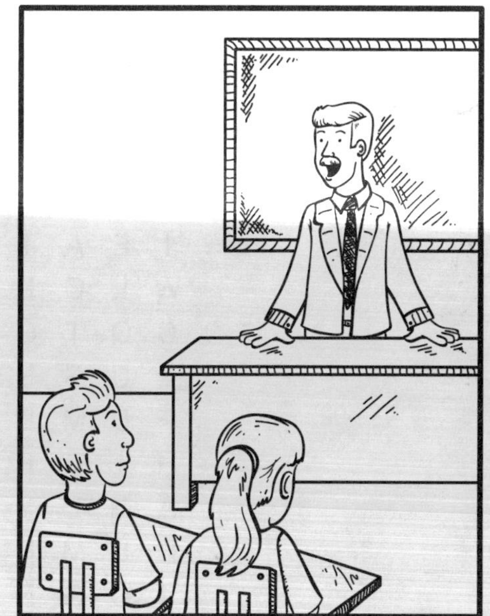

What Mr. Tuttle liked best about his classroom.

46.

APPLYING WHAT YOU KNOW

47. Mr. Nay was an avid swimmer and competed regularly in his age group. He had to withdraw from the last competition due to an infection of his ear. Antibiotics and analgesics were prescribed by the doctor. What is the medical term for his condition?

48. Mrs. Metheny loved the outdoors and spent a great deal of her spare time basking in the sun on the beach. Her physician suggested that she begin wearing sunglasses regularly when he noticed milky spots beginning to appear on Mrs. Metheny's lenses. What condition was Mrs. Metheny's physician trying to prevent?

49. Amanda repeatedly became ill with throat infections during her first few years of school. Lately, however, she has noticed that whenever she has a throat infection, her ears become very sore also. What might be the cause of this additional problem?

50. Julius was hit in the nose with a baseball during practice. His sense of smell was temporarily gone. What nerve receptors were damaged during the injury?

51. WORD FIND

Can you find the 19 terms from this chapter in the box of letters? Words may be spelled top to bottom, bottom to top, right to left, left to right, or diagonally.

```
M E C H A N O R E C E P T O R
H R A T B Q I R T B N H M A E
P F T Y R O T C A F L O X R C
G U A Y I N A I H C A T S U E
G P R A C E R U M E N O P X P
I E A I P O Y B S E R P K D T
W L C P L Y N E Y K E I T O O
C Q T O I B R J B S F G L M R
Z U S R C L E O U J R M N N S
F D M E O H L Q T N A E Y I S
H I D P N D L A M A C N X S Z
A M L Y E S S E E D T T M Z H
D D M H S F E X A Y I S I I A
J C G N J T I S L P O G U V J
P H G Y A K H S U C N I S G A
```

Cataracts	Gustatory	Presbyopia
Cerumen	Hyperopia	Receptors
Cochlea	Incus	Refraction
Cones	Mechanoreceptor	Rods
Conjunctiva	Olfactory	Senses
Eustachian	Papillae	
Eye	Photopigment	

DID YOU KNOW?

The human eye blinks an average of 4,200,000 times a year.

Our eyes are always the same size from birth, but our nose and ears never stop growing.

If your mouth was completely dry, you would not be able to distinguish the taste of anything.

THE SENSES

Fill in the crossword puzzle.

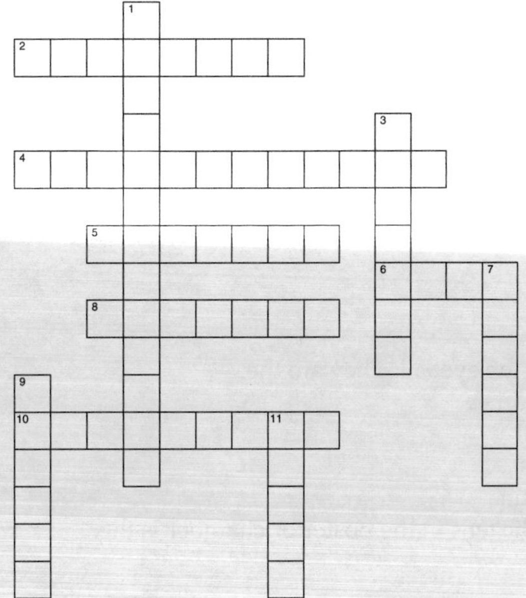

Across
2. Bones of the middle ear
4. Located in anterior cavity in front of lens (two words)
5. External ear
6. Transparent body behind pupil
8. Front part of this coat is the ciliary muscle and iris
10. Membranous labyrinth filled with this fluid

Down
1. Located in posterior cavity (two words)
3. Organ of Corti located here
7. White of the eye
9. Innermost layer of the eye
11. Hole in center of the iris

CHECK YOUR KNOWLEDGE

Multiple Choice

Circle the correct choice.

1. The Golgi tendon receptors and muscle spindles are important:
   A. Proprioceptors
   B. Photoreceptors
   C. Chemoreceptors
   D. None of the above
2. Another name for "farsightedness" is:
   A. Myopia
   B. Hyperopia
   C. Astigmatism
   D. None of the above
3. In addition to its role in hearing, the ear also functions as:
   A. The sense organ of equilibrium and balance
   B. A sense organ for chemoreceptors
   C. The sense organ for gustatory cells
   D. None of the above

4. The occipital lobe is responsible for:
   A. Interpretation of mechanoreceptors
   B. Interpretation of chemoreceptors
   C. Visual interpretation
   D. None of the above
5. Another name for the tympanic membrane is the:
   A. Ossicle
   B. Eardrum
   C. External auditory canal
   D. Oval window
6. The inner ear consists of three spaces in the temporal bone, assembled in a complex maze called the:
   A. Crista ampullaris
   B. Bony labyrinth
   C. Organ of Corti
   D. Ossicles
7. Three layers of tissue form the eyeball. They are the:
   A. Iris, conjunctiva, and cornea
   B. Choroid, iris, and pupil
   C. Retina, rods, and cones
   D. Sclera, choroid, and retina
8. The jellylike fluid behind the lens in the posterior chamber is the:
   A. Aqueous humor
   B. Vitreous humor
   C. Endolymph
   D. Perilymph
9. The Eustachian tube connects the throat with the:
   A. Tympanic membrane
   B. External ear
   C. Inner ear
   D. Middle ear
10. The receptors for night vision are the:
   A. Rods
   B. Cones
   C. Fovea centralis
   D. Chemoreceptors

True or False

Indicate whether the following statements are true (T) or false (F).

_____ 11. The sense organs are often classified as either general sense organs or special sense organs.

_____ 12. The cornea is sometimes spoken of as the "white of the eye."

_____ 13. Two involuntary muscles make up the front part of the choroid: the iris and the ciliary muscle.

_____ 14. When the lens becomes hard and loses its transparency, a condition called glaucoma occurs.

_____ 15. A laser surgery recently approved by the USFDA for hyperopia is laser thermal keratoplasty.

_____ 16. The optic disc is also known as the blind spot.

_____ 17. The malleus, incus, and stapes are also known as the ossicles.

_____ 18. A middle ear infection may also be referred to as otitis media.

_____ 19. The chemoreceptors of the taste buds are called gustatory cells.

_____ 20. Tears are formed in the lacrimal gland.

EYE

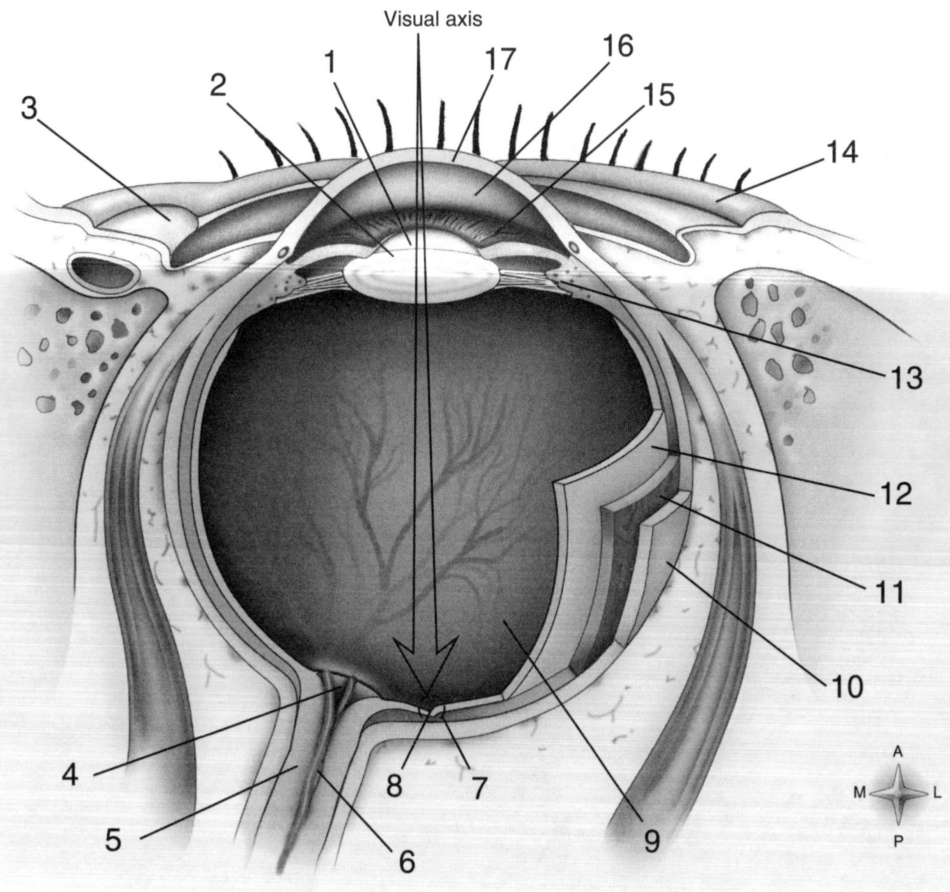

1. ______________________
2. ______________________
3. ______________________
4. ______________________
5. ______________________
6. ______________________
7. ______________________
8. ______________________
9. ______________________
10. ______________________
11. ______________________
12. ______________________
13. ______________________
14. ______________________
15. ______________________
16. ______________________
17. ______________________

EAR

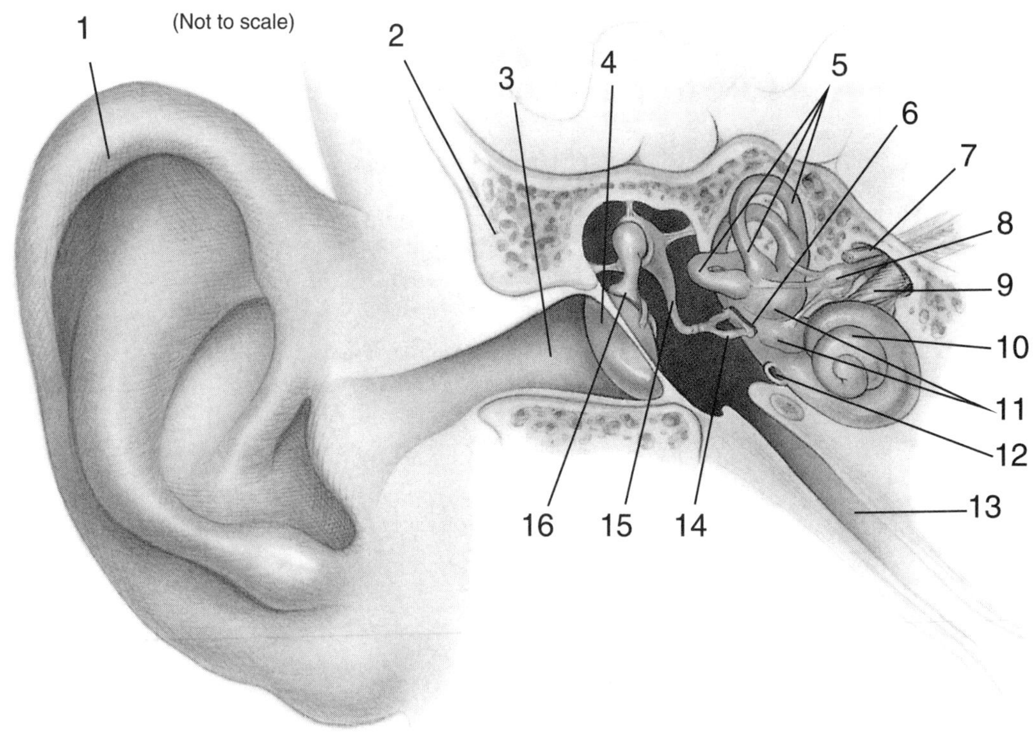

1. ______________________
2. ______________________
3. ______________________
4. ______________________
5. ______________________
6. ______________________
7. ______________________
8. ______________________
9. ______________________
10. ______________________
11. ______________________
12. ______________________
13. ______________________
14. ______________________
15. ______________________
16. ______________________

CHAPTER 10

The Endocrine System

The endocrine system has often been compared to a fine concert symphony. When all instruments are playing properly, the sound is melodious. If one instrument plays too loudly or too softly, however, it affects the overall quality of the performance.

The endocrine system is a ductless system that releases hormones into the bloodstream to help regulate body functions. The pituitary gland may be considered the conductor of the orchestra, as it stimulates many of the endocrine glands to secrete their powerful hormones. All hormones, whether stimulated in this manner or by other control mechanisms, are interdependent. A change in the level of one hormone may affect the level of many other hormones.

In addition to the endocrine glands, prostaglandins ("tissue hormones") are powerful substances similar to hormones that have been found in a variety of body tissues. These hormones are often produced in a tissue and diffuse only a short distance to act on cells within that area. Prostaglandins influence respiration, blood pressure, gastrointestinal secretions, and the reproductive system, and they may some day play an important role in the treatment of diseases such as hypertension, asthma, and ulcers.

The endocrine system is a system of communication and control. It differs from the nervous system in that hormones provide a slower, longer-lasting effect than do nerve stimuli and responses. Your understanding of the "system of hormones" will alert you to the mechanism of our emotions, responses to stress, growth, chemical balances, and many other body functions.

TOPICS FOR REVIEW

Before progressing to Chapter 11, you should be able to identify and locate the primary endocrine glands of the body. Your understanding should include the hormones that are produced by these glands and the method by which these secretions are regulated. Your study will conclude with the pathological conditions that result from the malfunctioning of this system.

MECHANISMS OF HORMONE ACTION REGULATION OF HORMONE SECRETION PROSTAGLANDINS

Match the term on the left with the proper selection on the right.

Group A

_____ 1. Pituitary
_____ 2. Parathyroids
_____ 3. Adrenals
_____ 4. Ovaries
_____ 5. Thymus

A. Pelvic cavity
B. Mediastinum
C. Neck
D. Cranial cavity
E. Abdominal cavity

Group B

_____ 6. Negative feedback
_____ 7. Tissue hormones
_____ 8. Second messenger
_____ 9. Exocrine glands
_____ 10. Target organ cells

A. Cyclic AMP is an example of one
B. Respond to a particular hormone
C. Prostaglandins
D. Discharge secretions into ducts
E. Specialized homeostatic mechanism that regulates release of hormones

Fill in the blanks.

Nonsteroid hormones serve as (11) __________ ________________ providing communication between (12) ____________ and (13) _________ _________. Another molecule such as (14) ________ ___________ then acts as the (15) ___________ ___________ providing (16) ____________________ within a hormone's (17) _______________ ____________.

If you have had difficulty with this section, review pages 250-258.

PITUITARY GLAND HYPOTHALAMUS

Circle the correct answer.

18. The pituitary gland lies in the ___________________ bone.
    A. Ethmoid
    B. Sphenoid
    C. Temporal
    D. Frontal
    E. Occipital

19. Which one of the following structures would *not* be stimulated by a tropic hormone from the anterior pituitary?
    A. Ovaries
    B. Testes
    C. Thyroid
    D. Adrenals
    E. Uterus

20. Which one of the following is *not* a function of FSH?
    A. Stimulates the growth of follicles
    B. Stimulates the production of estrogens
    C. Stimulates the growth of seminiferous tubules
    D. Stimulates the interstitial cells of the testes

21. Which one of the following is *not* a function of LH?
    A. Stimulates maturation of a developing follicle
    B. Stimulates the production of estrogens
    C. Stimulates the formation of a corpus luteum
    D. Stimulates sperm cells to mature in the male
    E. Causes ovulation

22. Which one of the following is *not* a function of GH?
    A. Increases glucose catabolism
    B. Increases fat catabolism
    C. Speeds up the movement of amino acids into cells from the bloodstream
    D. All of the above are functions of GH

23. Which one of the following hormones is *not* released by the anterior pituitary gland?
    A. ACTH
    B. TSH
    C. ADH
    D. FSH
    E. LH

24. Which one of the following is *not* a function of prolactin?
    A. Stimulates breast development during pregnancy
    B. Stimulates milk secretion after delivery
    C. Causes the release of milk from glandular cells of the breast
    D. All of the above are functions of prolactin

25. The anterior pituitary gland secretes:
    A. Eight major hormones
    B. Tropic hormones that stimulate other endocrine glands to grow and secrete
    C. ADH
    D. Oxytocin

26. TSH acts on the:
    A. Thyroid
    B. Thymus
    C. Pineal
    D. Testes

27. ACTH stimulates the:
    A. Adrenal cortex
    B. Adrenal medulla
    C. Hypothalamus
    D. Ovaries

28. Which hormone is secreted by the posterior pituitary gland?
    A. MSH
    B. LH
    C. GH
    D. ADH

29. ADH serves the body by:
    A. Initiating labor
    B. Accelerating water reabsorption from urine into the blood
    C. Stimulating the pineal gland
    D. Regulating the calcium/phosphorus levels in the blood

30. What disease is caused by hyposecretion of ADH?
    A. Diabetes insipidus
    B. Diabetes mellitus
    C. Acromegaly
    D. Myxedema

31. The actual production of ADH and oxytocin takes place in which area?
    A. Anterior pituitary
    B. Posterior pituitary
    C. Hypothalamus
    D. Pineal

32. Inhibiting hormones are produced by the:
    A. Anterior pituitary
    B. Posterior pituitary
    C. Hypothalamus
    D. Pineal

Select the correct term from the choices given and write the letter in the answer blank.

(A) Anterior pituitary (B) Posterior pituitary (C) Hypothalamus

_____ 33. Adenohypophysis

_____ 34. Neurohypophysis

_____ 35. Induced labor

_____ 36. Appetite

_____ 37. Acromegaly

_____ 38. Body temperature

_____ 39. Sex hormones

_____ 40. Tropic hormones

_____ 41. Gigantism

_____ 42. Releasing hormones

If you have had difficulty with this section, review pages 258-261.

THYROID GLAND
PARATHYROID GLANDS

Circle the correct answer.

43. The thyroid gland lies (above or below) the larynx.
44. The thyroid gland secretes (calcitonin or glucagon).
45. For thyroxine to be produced in adequate amounts, the diet must contain sufficient (calcium or iodine).
46. Most endocrine glands (do or do not) store their hormones.
47. Colloid is a storage medium for the (thyroid or parathyroid) hormone.
48. Calcitonin (increases or decreases) the concentration of calcium in the blood.
49. Simple goiter results from (hyperthyroidism or hypothyroidism).
50. Hyposecretion of thyroid hormones during the formative years leads to (cretinism or myxedema).
51. The parathyroid glands secrete the hormone (PTH or PTA).
52. Parathyroid hormone tends to (increase or decrease) the concentration of calcium in the blood.

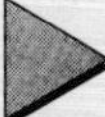

If you have had difficulty with this section, review pages 261-264.

ADRENAL GLANDS

Fill in the blanks.

53. The adrenal gland is actually two separate endocrine glands, the ____________ ____________ and the ____________ ____________.
54. Hormones secreted by the adrenal cortex are known as ______________.
55. The outer zone of the adrenal cortex secretes ________________.
56. The middle zone secretes ______________.
57. The innermost zone secretes ____________ ______________.
58. Glucocorticoids act in several ways to increase ______________.
59. Glucocorticoids also play an essential part in maintaining ____________ ____________.
60. The adrenal medulla secretes the hormones ______________ and ______________.
61. The adrenal medulla may help the body resist ______________.
62. Deficiency or hyposecretion of adrenal cortex hormones results in a condition called ________ ________.

Select the correct term from the choices given and write the letter in the answer blank.

(A) Adrenal cortex (B) Adrenal medulla

_____ 63. Mineralocorticoids

_____ 64. Anti-immunity

_____ 65. Adrenaline

_____ 66. Cushing's syndrome

_____ 67. "Fight or flight" response

_____ 68. Aldosterone

_____ 69. Androgens

If you have had difficulty with this section, review pages 263-268.

PANCREATIC ISLETS, SEX GLANDS, THYMUS, PLACENTA, PINEAL GLAND

Circle the term that does not *belong.*

70. Alpha cells	Glucagon	Beta cells	Glycogenolysis
71. Insulin	Glucagon	Beta cells	Diabetes mellitus
72. Estrogens	Progesterone	Corpus luteum	Thymosin
73. Chorion	Interstitial cells	Testosterone	Semen
74. Immune system	Mediastinum	Aldosterone	Thymosin
75. Pregnancy	ACTH	Estrogen	Chorion
76. Melatonin	Menstruation	"Third eye"	Semen

Match the term on the left with the proper selection on the right.

Group A

_____ 77. Alpha cells A. Estrogen
_____ 78. Beta cells B. Progesterone
_____ 79. Corpus luteum C. Insulin
_____ 80. Interstitial cells D. Testosterone
_____ 81. Ovarian follicles E. Glucagon

Group B

_____ 82. Placenta A. Melatonin
_____ 83. Pineal B. ANH
_____ 84. Heart atria C. Testosterone
_____ 85. Testes D. Thymosin
_____ 86. Thymus E. Chorionic gonadotropins

If you have had difficulty with this section, review pages 268-272.

UNSCRAMBLE THE WORDS

Take the circled letters, unscramble them, and fill in the statement.

87. **ROODIITSCC**

88. **SIUISERD**

89. **UOOOTDCSIILRCCG**

90. **RIODSTES**

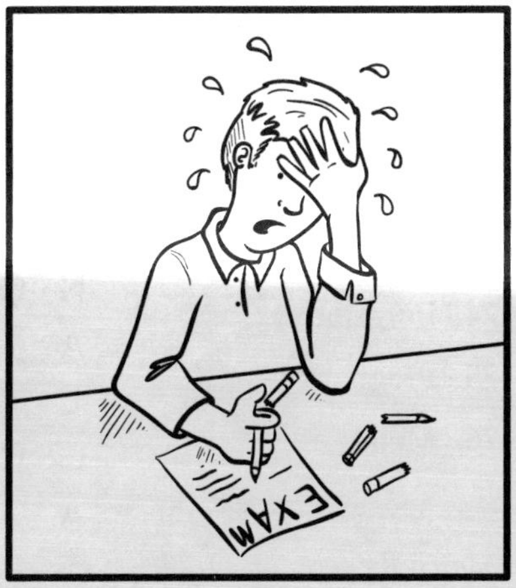

Why Billy didn't like to take exams.

91.

APPLYING WHAT YOU KNOW

92. Mrs. Fortner made a routine visit to her physician last week. When the laboratory results came back, the report indicated a high level of chorionic gonadotropin in her urine. What did this mean to Mrs. Fortner?

93. Mrs. Wilcox noticed that her daughter was beginning to take on some of the secondary sex characteristics of a male. The pediatrician diagnosed the condition as a tumor of an endocrine gland. Where specifically was the tumor located?

94. Mrs. Florez was pregnant and was 2 weeks past her due date. Her doctor suggested that she enter the hospital and said he would induce labor. What hormone will he give Mrs. Florez?

95. WORD FIND

Can you find the 16 terms from the chapter in the box of letters? Words may be spelled top to bottom, bottom to top, right to left, left to right, or diagonally.

S S I S E R U I D M E S I T W
N D N X E B A M E D E X Y M I
I I G O N R S G X T I I Y V B
D O M S I N I T E R C C U Q D
N C X S R T N B O T V M Y O M
A I M E C L A C R E P Y H I X
L T Y R O I E Z Q R T J V K F
G R E T D P S N I L D J M X N
A O O S N I D K I N K S P P O
T C P R E T I O G R I F M X G
S L M H Y P O G L Y C E M I A
O A J L H O R M O N E O T G C
R C E L T S E L C N P N X U U
P I O S W R T X C G U L O E L
G G V Y H M S H Y K A K N Q G

Corticoids	Glucagon	Myxedema
Cretinism	Goiter	Prostaglandins
Diabetes	Hormone	Steroids
Diuresis	Hypercalcemia	Stress
Endocrine	Hypoglycemia	
Exocrine	Luteinization	

DID YOU KNOW?

The pituitary weighs little more than a small paper clip.

The total daily output of the pituitary gland is less than 1/1,000,000 of a gram, yet this small amount is responsible for stimulating the majority of all endocrine functions.

THE ENDOCRINE SYSTEM

Fill in the crossword puzzle.

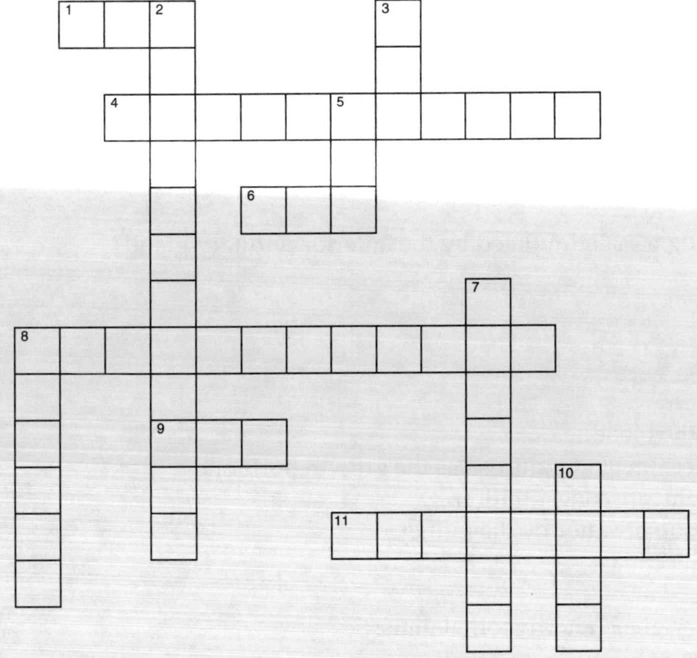

Across
1. Secreted by cells in the walls of the heart's atria
4. Adrenal medulla
6. Estrogens
8. Converts amino acids to glucose
9. Melanin
11. Labor

Down
2. Hypersecretion of insulin
3. Antagonist to diuresis
5. Increases calcium concentration
7. Hyposecretion of islets of Langerhans (one word)
8. Hyposecretion of thyroid
10. Adrenal cortex

CHECK YOUR KNOWLEDGE

Multiple Choice

Circle the correct answer.

1. All of the following are included in the endocrine system *except*:
   A. Exocrine glands
   B. Steroid hormones
   C. Nonsteroid hormones
   D. All of the above are included in the endocrine system

2. The luteinizing hormone (LH) stimulates:
   A. Breast development during pregnancy
   B. The development of ovarian follicles
   C. Maturation of ovarian follicle and triggers ovulation
   D. Seminiferous tubules of testes to grow and produce sperm

3. Prostaglandins or tissue hormones influence:
   A. Respiration
   B. Gastrointestinal secretions
   C. Blood pressure
   D. All of the above

4. Which of the following is *not* stimulated by the anterior pituitary gland?
   A. TSH
   B. ACTH
   C. ADH
   D. FSH

5. Too much insulin in the blood:
   A. Has the same effect on blood glucose as the growth hormone
   B. Increases blood glucose concentration
   C. Stimulates retention of water by the kidneys
   D. Produces hypoglycemia

6. The posterior pituitary gland and hypothalamus:
   A. Release two hormones
   B. Produce substances called releasing and inhibiting hormones
   C. Cause the glandular cells of the breast to release milk into ducts for nursing a baby
   D. All of the above

7. In addition to producing thyroid hormones, the thyroid gland also secretes:
   A. Hydrocortisone
   B. Calcitonin
   C. Aldosterone
   D. Glucagon

8. The adrenal medulla produces hormones that are:
   A. Not essential for life
   B. Helpful in responding to stress
   C. Responsible for the "fight or flight" response
   D. All of the above

9. The pineal gland produces several hormones in small quantities, with the most significant being:
   A. ANH
   B. Leptin
   C. Chorionic gonadotropins
   D. Melatonin

10. What plays a critical role in the body's defenses against infections?
    A. Pancreas
    B. Thymus
    C. Pineal body
    D. Thyroid

MATCHING

Select the most correct answer from column B for each statement in column A. (Only one answer is correct.)

Column A	Column B
_____ 11. Steroid hormones	A. Pancreas
_____ 12. Positive feedback	B. Adrenal cortex
_____ 13. Tropic hormones	C. Progesterone
_____ 14. Myxedema	D. Diabetes mellitus
_____ 15. Glucocorticoids	E. "Third eye"
_____ 16. Aldosterone	F. Mineralocorticoid
_____ 17. Islets of Langerhans	G. Occurs during labor
_____ 18. Glycosuria	H. Anterior pituitary
_____ 19. Pineal gland	I. Thyroid gland
_____ 20. Corpus luteum	J. Lipid soluble

ENDOCRINE GLANDS

1. ______________________________
2. ______________________________
3. ______________________________
4. ______________________________
5. ______________________________
6. ______________________________
7. ______________________________
8. ______________________________
9. ______________________________
10. ______________________________

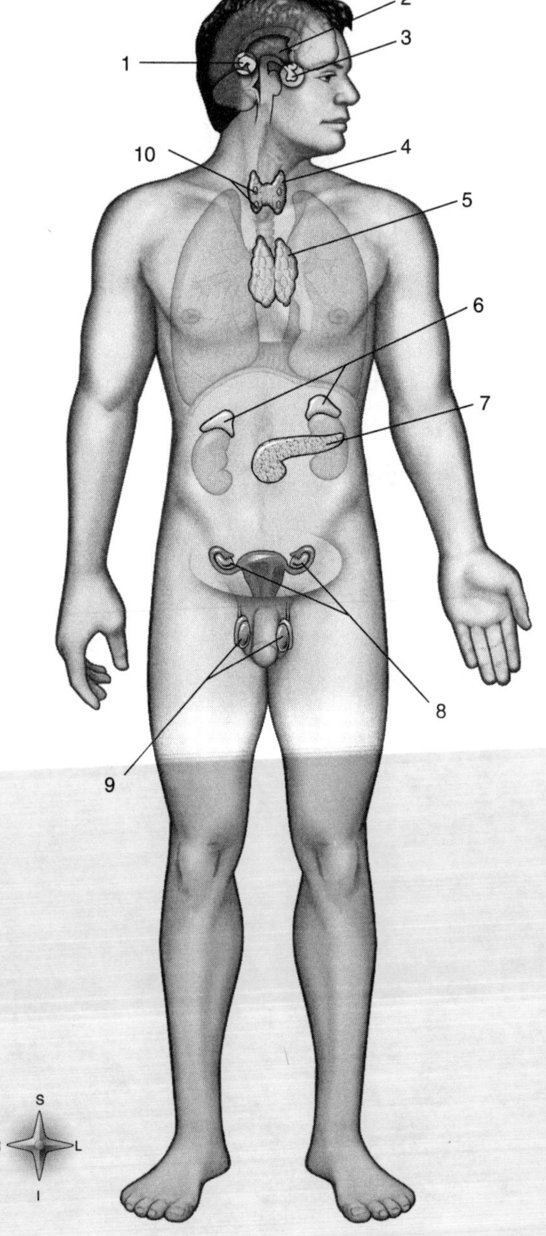

70. WORD FIND

Can you find 15 terms from this chapter in the box of letters? Words may be spelled t om to top, right to left, left to right, or diagonally.

```
Y H Y S I S O B M O R H T A
L A C I L I B M U O A Y N I
E E S Y S T E M I C C G D E
M V E N U L E D D C I X M D
E Y M U I R T A R N L E C G Y
N O I T A Z I R A L O P E D N
U D L A T R O P C I T A P E H
S I U K M U E T O E S L U P U
R P N F Y C B E D R A L Z P J
D S A H T I T V N L I I B D W
Q U R O I V A Q E O D A K R K
K C R M P G A I G N D D Z Y J
Y I Y R I N E A F Z L Q S P X
S R M I C C Q O A W U N H O K
P T A V H H Z L H I J J X K Z
```

Angina pectoris	ECG	Systemic
Apex	Endocardium	Thrombosis
Atrium	Hepatic portal	Tricuspid
Depolarization	Pulse	Umbilical
Diastolic	Semilunar	Venule

DID YOU KNOW?

Your heart pumps more than 5 quarts of blood every minute or 2,000 gallor a d

Every pound of excess fat contains some 200 miles of additional capillaries o p blood thro each minute.

If laid out in a straight line, the average adult's circulatory system would b n y 60,000 mil ong—enough to circle the earth 2.5 times!

CIRCULATORY SYSTEM

Fill in the crossword puzzle.

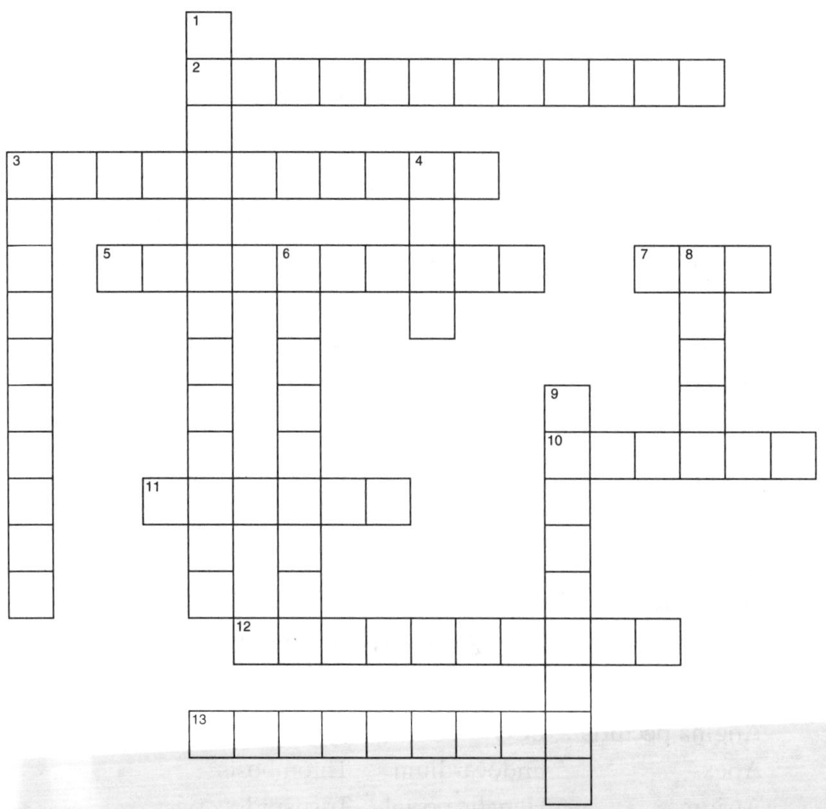

Across

2. Inflammation of the lining of the heart
3. Bicuspid valve (2 words)
5. Inner layer of pericardium
7. Cardiopulmonary resuscitation (abbreviation)
10. Carries blood away from the heart
11. Upper chamber of heart
12. Lower chambers of the heart
13. SA node

Down

1. Unique blood circulation through the liver (2 words)
3. Muscular layer of the heart
4. Carries blood to the heart
6. Tiny artery
8. Heart rate
9. Carries blood from arterioles into venules

PRINCIPAL ARTERIES OF THE BODY

1. ________________
2. ________________
3. ________________
4. ________________
5. ________________
6. ________________
7. ________________
8. ________________
9. ________________
10. ________________
11. ________________
12. ________________
13. ________________
14. ________________
15. ________________
16. ________________
17. ________________
18. ________________
19. ________________
20. ________________
21. ________________
22. ________________
23. ________________
24. ________________
25. ________________
26. ________________
27. ________________
28. ________________
29. ________________
30. ________________

PRINCIPAL VEINS OF THE BODY

1. ______________________
2. ______________________
3. ______________________
4. ______________________
5. ______________________
6. ______________________
7. ______________________
8. ______________________
9. ______________________
10. ______________________
11. ______________________
12. ______________________
13. ______________________
14. ______________________
15. ______________________
16. ______________________
17. ______________________
18. ______________________
19. ______________________
20. ______________________
21. ______________________
22. ______________________
23. ______________________
24. ______________________
25. ______________________
26. ______________________
27. ______________________
28. ______________________
29. ______________________
30. ______________________
31. ______________________
32. ______________________
33. ______________________
34. ______________________

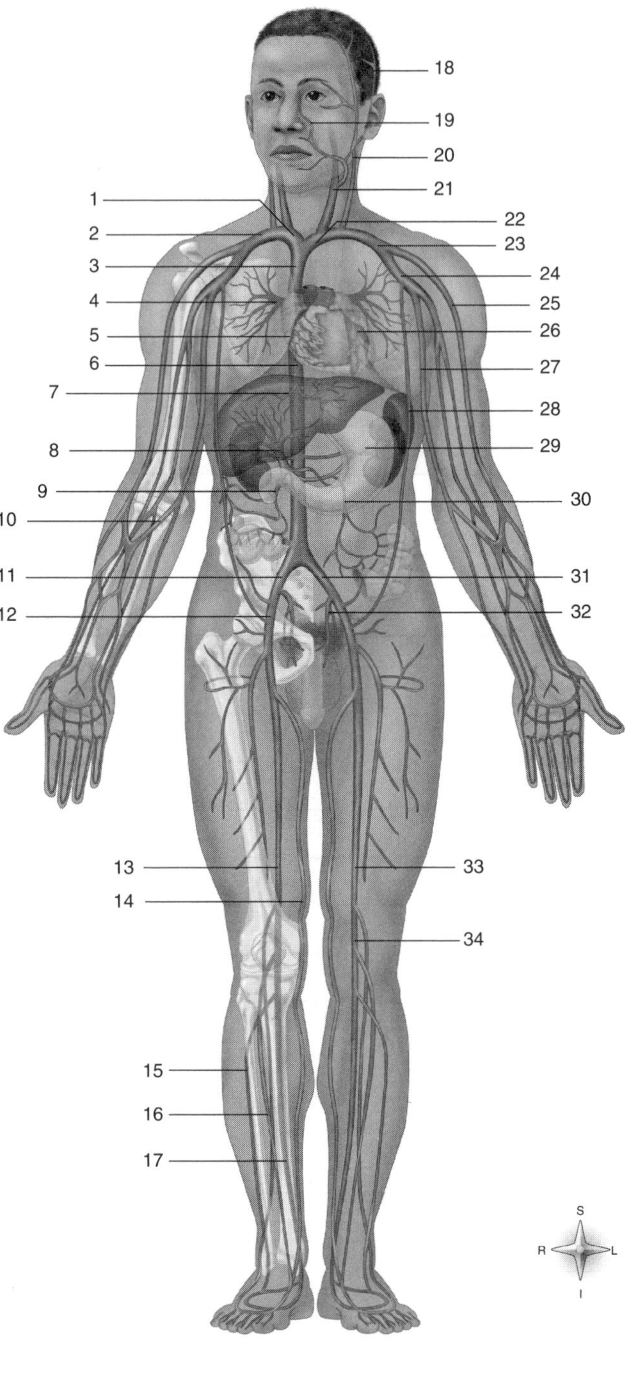

CHAPTER 13

The Lymphatic System and Immunity

The lymphatic system is similar to the circulatory system. Lymph, like blood, flows through an elaborate route of vessels. In addition to lymphatic vessels, the lymphatic system consists of lymph nodes, lymph, and the spleen. Unlike the circulatory system, the lymphatic vessels do not form a closed circuit. Lymph flows only once through the vessels before draining into the general blood circulation. This system is a filtering mechanism for microorganisms and serves as a protective device against foreign invaders, such as cancer.

The immune system is the armed forces division of the body. Ready to attack at a moment's notice, the immune system defends us against the major enemies of the body: microorganisms, foreign transplanted tissue cells, and our own cells that have turned malignant.

The most numerous cells of the immune system are the lymphocytes. These cells circulate in the body's fluids seeking invading organisms and destroying them with powerful lymphotoxins, lymphokines, or antibodies.

Phagocytes, another large group of immune system cells, assist with the destruction of foreign invaders by a process known as phagocytosis. Neutrophils, monocytes, and connective tissue cells called macrophages use this process to surround unwanted microorganisms, ingest and digest them, and render them harmless to the body.

Another weapon that the immune system possesses is complement. Normally a group of inactive enzymes present in the blood, complement can be activated to kill invading cells by drilling holes in their cytoplasmic membranes allowing fluid to enter the cell until it bursts.

Your review of this chapter will give you an understanding of how the body defends itself from the daily invasion of destructive substances.

TOPICS FOR REVIEW

Before progressing to Chapter 14 you should familiarize yourself with the functions of the lymphatic system, the immune system, and the major structures that make up these systems. Your review should include knowledge of lymphatic vessels, lymph nodes, lymph, antibodies, complement, and the development of B and T cells. Your study should conclude with an understanding of the differences in humoral and cell-mediated immunity.

THE LYMPHATIC SYSTEM

Fill in the blanks.

1. ___________________ is a specialized fluid formed in the tissue spaces that will be transported by way of specialized vessels to eventually reenter the circulatory system.
2. Blood plasma that has filtered out of capillaries into microscopic spaces between cells is called ______________ __________________.
3. The network of tiny blind-ended tubes distributed in the tissue spaces is called __________ __________.
4. Lymph eventually empties into two terminal vessels called the ___________ _____________ _______________ and the _____________ ________________.
5. The thoracic duct has an enlarged pouchlike structure called the _____________ ________________.
6. Lymph is filtered by moving through _____________ _______________, located in clusters along the pathway of lymphatic vessels.
7. Lymph enters the node through four _____________________ lymph vessels.
8. Lymph exits from the node through a single ______________ lymph vessel.

If you have had difficulty with this section, review pages 336-341.

THYMUS, TONSILS, SPLEEN

Select the correct term from the options given and write the letter in the answer blank.

(A) Thymus (B) Tonsils (C) Spleen

_____ 9. Palatine, pharyngeal, and lingual are examples
_____ 10. Largest lymphoid organ in the body
_____ 11. Destroys worn-out red blood cells
_____ 12. Located in the mediastinum
_____ 13. Serves as a reservoir for blood
_____ 14. T-lymphocytes
_____ 15. Largest at puberty

If you have had difficulty with this section, review pages 341-344.

THE IMMUNE SYSTEM

Match the term on the left with the proper selection on the right.

_____ 16. Nonspecific immunity
_____ 17. Mother's milk
_____ 18. Specific immunity
_____ 19. Artificial passive immunity
_____ 20. Immunization

A. Natural passive immunity
B. Injection of antibodies
C. General protection
D. Artificial active exposure
E. Adaptive immunity

If you have had difficulty with this section, review pages 344-346.

IMMUNE SYSTEM MOLECULES

Choose the term that applies to each of the following descriptions. Write the letter for the term in the appropriate answer blank.

A. Antibodies
B. Antigen
C. Allergy
D. Anaphylactic shock
E. Monoclonal
F. Complement cascade
G. Complement
H. Humoral immunity
I. Combining site
J. hCG

_____ 21. Hypersensitivity of the immune system to harmless antigens

_____ 22. Life-threatening allergic reaction

_____ 23. Type of very specific antibodies produced from a population of identical cells

_____ 24. Protein compounds normally present in the body

_____ 25. Also known as antibody-mediated immunity

_____ 26. Combines with antibody to produce humoral immunity

_____ 27. Antibody

_____ 28. Process of changing molecule shape slightly to expose binding sites

_____ 29. Pregnancy test kits

_____ 30. Inactive proteins in blood

Circle the one that does not *belong.*

31. Antibody	Allergy	Protein compound	Combining site
32. Antigen	Invading cells	Foreign protein	Complement
33. Monoclonal	Antibodies	Antigen	Specific
34. Allergy	Complement	Anaphylactic shock	Antigen
35. Monoclonal	14	Complement	Proteins

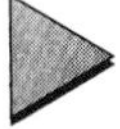
If you have had difficulty with this section, review pages 346-348.

IMMUNE SYSTEM CELLS

Multiple Choice

Circle the correct answer.

36. The most numerous cells of the immune system are the:
    A. Monocytes
    B. Eosinophils
    C. Neutrophils
    D. Lymphocytes
    E. Complement

37. Which of the terms listed below occurs third in the immune process?
    A. Plasma cells
    B. Stem cells
    C. Antibodies
    D. Activated B cells
    E. Immature B cells

38. Which one of the terms listed below occurs last in the immune process?
    A. Plasma cells
    B. Stem cells
    C. Antibodies
    D. Activated B cells
    E. Immature B cells

39. Moderate exercise has been found to:
    A. Decrease white blood cells
    B. Increase white blood cells
    C. Decrease platelets
    D. Decrease red blood cells

40. Which one of the following is part of the cell membrane of B cells?
    A. Complement
    B. Antigens
    C. Antibodies
    D. Epitopes
    E. None of the above

41. Immature B cells have:
    A. Four types of defense mechanisms on their cell membrane
    B. Several kinds of defense mechanisms on their cell membrane
    C. One specific kind of defense mechanism on their cell membrane
    D. No defense mechanisms on their cell membrane

42. Development of an immature B cell depends on the B cell coming in contact with:
    A. Complement
    B. Antibodies
    C. Lymphotoxins
    D. Lymphokines
    E. Antigens

43. The kind of cell that produces large numbers of antibodies is the:
    A. B cell
    B. Stem cell
    C. T cell
    D. Memory cell
    E. Plasma cell

44. Just one of these short-lived cells that make antibodies can produce ______________ of them per second.
    A. 20
    B. 200
    C. 2,000
    D. 20,000

45. Which of the following statements is *not* true of memory cells?
    A. They produce large numbers of antibodies.
    B. They are found in lymph nodes.
    C. They develop into plasma cells.
    D. They can react with antigens.
    E. All of the above are true of memory cells.

46. T cell development begins in the:
    A. Lymph nodes
    B. Liver
    C. Pancreas
    D. Spleen
    E. Thymus

47. Human immunodeficiency virus (HIV) has its most obvious effects in:
    A. B cells
    B. Stem cells
    C. Plasma cells
    D. T cells

48. Interferon:
    A. Is produced by T cells within hours after infection by a virus
    B. Decreases the severity of many virus-related diseases
    C. Shows promise as an anticancer agent
    D. Has been shown to be effective in treating breast cancer
    E. All of the above

49. B cells function indirectly to produce:
    A. Humoral immunity
    B. Cell-mediated immunity
    C. Lymphotoxins
    D. Lymphokines

50. T cells function to produce:
    A. Humoral immunity
    B. Cell-mediated immunity
    C. Antibodies
    D. Memory cells

Fill in the blanks.

51. The first stage of development for B cells is called the ________________ ________________.
52. The second stage of B cell development changes an immature B cell into a(n) ________________ ________________ ________________.
53. ________________ ________________ secrete copious amounts of antibody into the blood—nearly 2,000 antibody molecules for every second they live.
54. T cells are lymphocytes that have undergone their first stage of development in the ________________ ________________.
55. ________________ blocks HIV's ability to reproduce within infected cells.
56. ________________ is a disease caused by a retrovirus that enters the bloodstream and integrates into the DNA of T cell lymphocytes.
57. Like many viruses, such as the common cold, HIV changes rapidly so the development of a ________________ may not occur for several years.

If you have had difficulty with this section, review pages 348-355.

UNSCRAMBLE THE WORDS

Take the circled letters, unscramble them, and fill in the statement.

58. **NTCMPEOLEM**

59. **MTMYIUNI**

60. **OENCLS**

61. **FNROERTENI**

What the student was praying for the night before exams.

62.

APPLYING WHAT YOU KNOW

63. Two-year old baby Metcalfe was exposed to chickenpox. He had been a particularly sickly child and so the doctor decided to give him a dose of interferon. What effect was the physician hoping for in baby Metcalfe's case?

64. Marcia was an intravenous drug user. She was recently diagnosed with Kaposi's sarcoma. What is another possible diagnosis?

65. Baby Phelps was born without a thymus gland. Immediate plans were made for a transplant to be performed. In the meantime, baby Phelps was placed in strict isolation. Why was this done?

66. WORD FIND

Can you find 14 terms from the chapter in the box of letters? Words may be spelled top to bottom, bottom to top, right to left, left to right, or diagonally.

```
I N F L A M M A T O R Y F C G
Q N L O Y Z O C C P A O F S X
M W T A A M N J X Q K R N P H
U R L E R M P X B R U I A L C
C M A C R O P H A G E I E D Z
X M N D K F M N O T U C R N M
A E O R E Z E U O C F B Y E B
Y P L E B G G R H T Y T S E D
Y S C R I S P J O E I T M L A
Z M O T J X E T O N A E E P X
T O N S I L S S U M Y H T S Y
W A O C J N I M W K O Z E N D
D W M K W R M O I P S H Y B G
F H W U J I Z F V D Z L Y T X
```

Acquired	Interferon	Proteins
Antigen	Lymph	Spleen
Humoral	Lymphocytes	Thymus
Immunity	Macrophage	Tonsils
Inflammatory	Monoclonal	

DID YOU KNOW?

There are more living organisms on the skin of a single human being than there are human beings on the surface of the earth.

According to the Centers for Disease Control (CDC), 18 million courses of antibiotics are prescribed for the common cold in the United States per year. Research show that colds are caused by viruses. Fifty million unnecessary antibiotics are prescribed for viral respiratory infections.

LYMPH AND IMMUNITY

Fill in the crossword puzzle.

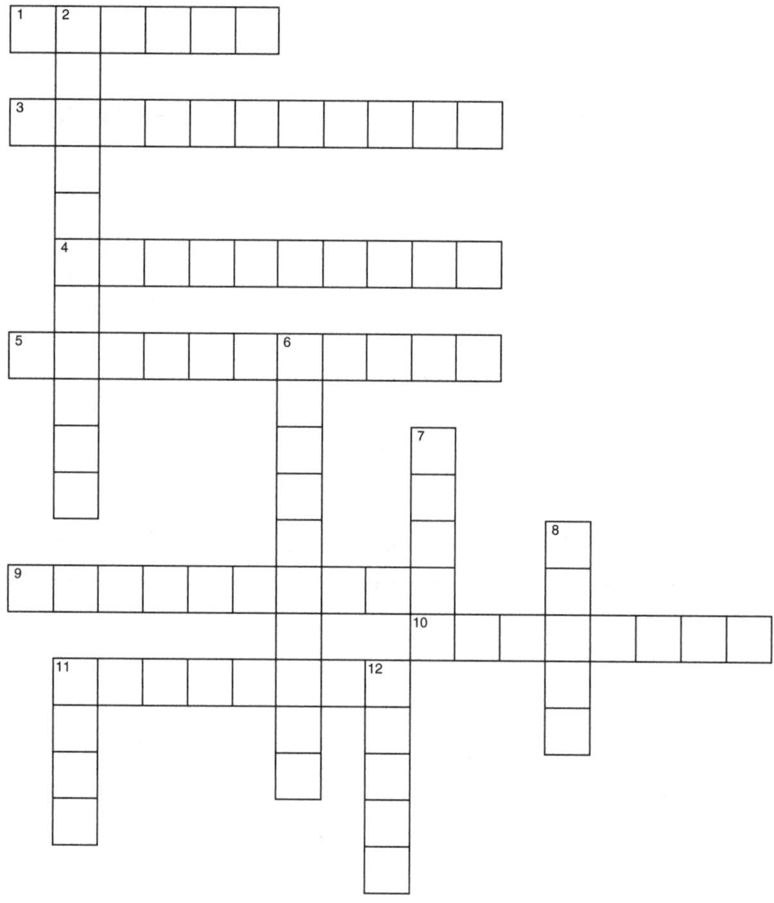

Across

1. Largest lymphoid organ in the body
3. Connective tissue cells that are phagocytes
4. Protein compounds normally present in the body
5. Remain in reserve then turn into plasma cells when needed (2 words)
9. Synthetically produced to fight certain diseases
10. Lymph exits the node through this lymph vessel
11. Lymph enters the node through these lymph vessels

Down

2. Secretes a copious amount of antibodies into the blood (2 words)
6. Inactive proteins
7. Family of identical cells descended from one cell
8. Type of lymphocyte (humoral immunity—2 words)
11. Immune deficiency disorder
12. Type of lymphocyte (cell-mediated immunity—2 words)

CHECK YOUR KNOWLEDGE

Multiple Choice

Circle the correct answer.

1. Which of the following is true about both lymphatic and blood capillaries?
   A. Both types of vessels are microscopic and are formed from sheets of endothelium.
   B. The movement and route of blood and lymph are identical.
   C. Both lymph and blood terminate into the same veins.
   D. All of the above are true.

2. The spleen:
   A. Is the largest lymphoid organ in the body
   B. Has a limited blood supply
   C. Is located in the upper right quadrant of the abdomen lateral to the stomach
   D. All of the above

3. Lymph nodes are responsible for:
   A. Defense
   B. White blood cell formation
   C. Biological filtration
   D. All of the above

4. Which of the following is *not* true regarding lymph vessels?
   A. Lymph enters the node through four afferent lymph vessels.
   B. Lymph exits the node through four efferent vessels.
   C. Once lymph enters the node, it "percolates" slowly through spaces called sinuses.
   D. Lymph from the breast drains into many different and widely placed nodes.

5. The thymus is:
   A. Largest at puberty
   B. A source of lymphocytes before birth
   C. Replaced by a process call involution
   D. All of the above

6. Which of the following is *not* an example of tonsils?
   A. Palatine
   B. Humoral
   C. Pharyngeal
   D. Lingual

7. Active immunity occurs when:
   A. Immunity to a disease that has developed in another individual is transferred to someone not previously immune
   B. An infant receives antibodies in her mother's milk
   C. Immunity is inherited
   D. A vaccination confers immunity

8. The function of T cells is to:
   A. Produce cell-mediated immunity
   B. Kill invading cells by releasing a substance that poisons cells
   C. Release chemicals that attract and activate macrophages to kill cells by phagocytosis
   D. All of the above

9. Which of the following is an example of nonspecific immunity?
   A. Skin
   B. Tears and mucous
   C. Inflammation
   D. All of the above

10. In general, antibodies produce __________ immunity.
   A. Complement
   B. Phagocytic
   C. Humoral
   D. Inherited

Matching

Select the most correct answer from column B for each statement in column A. (Only one answer is correct.)

Column A	Column B
_____ 11. Lymph vessel	A. Humoral
_____ 12. Thymus	B. Allergy
_____ 13. Nonspecific immunity	C. Interferon
_____ 14. Specific immunity	D. T-cells
_____ 15. Protein compounds in the body	E. Efferent
_____ 16. Antigen hypersensitivity	F. Macrophages
_____ 17. Antibody-mediated immunity	G. Antibodies
_____ 18. Monoclonal antibodies	H. Adaptive immunity
_____ 19. Synthetic treatment for viral infections	I. Phagocytosis
_____ 20. Kupffer's cells	J. Pregnancy test kits

PRINCIPAL ORGANS OF THE LYMPHATIC SYSTEM

1. ____________________
2. ____________________
3. ____________________
4. ____________________
5. ____________________
6. ____________________
7. ____________________
8. ____________________
9. ____________________
10. ____________________
11. ____________________
12. ____________________

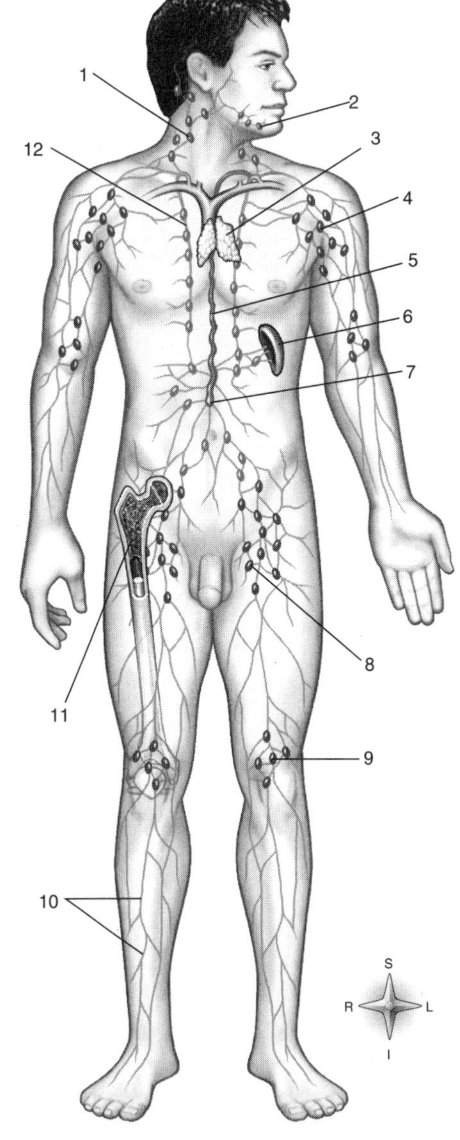

CHAPTER 14

The Respiratory System

As you sit reviewing this system, your body needs 16 quarts of air per minute. Walking requires 24 quarts of air per minute, and running requires 50 quarts per minute. The respiratory system provides the air necessary for you to perform your daily activities and eliminates the waste gases from the air that you breathe. Take a deep breath, and think of the air as entering some 250 million tiny air sacs similar in appearance to clusters of grapes. These microscopic air sacs expand to let air in and contract to force it out. These tiny sacs, alveoli, are the functioning units of the respiratory system. They provide the necessary volume of oxygen and eliminate carbon dioxide 24 hours a day.

Air enters either through the mouth or the nasal cavity. It next passes through the pharynx and past the epiglottis, then through the glottis and the rest of the larynx. It then continues down the trachea, into the bronchi to the bronchioles, and finally through the alveoli. The reverse occurs for expelled air.

The exchange of gases between air in the lungs and in the blood is known as external respiration. The exchange of gases that occurs between the blood and the cells of the body is known as internal respiration. By constantly supplying adequate oxygen and by removing carbon dioxide as it forms, the respiratory system helps to maintain an environment conducive to maximum cell efficiency.

Your review of this system is necessary to provide you with an understanding of this essential homeostatic mechanism.

TOPICS FOR REVIEW

Before progressing to Chapter 15, you should have an understanding of the structure and function of the organs of the respiratory system. Your review should include knowledge of the mechanisms responsible for both internal and external respiration. Your study should conclude with a knowledge of the volumes of air exchanged in pulmonary ventilation and an understanding of how respiration is regulated.

STRUCTURAL PLAN
RESPIRATORY TRACTS
RESPIRATORY MUCOSA

Match the term with the definition.

A. Diffusion
B. Respiratory membrane
C. Alveoli
D. URI
E. Respiration
F. Respiratory mucosa
G. Upper respiratory tract
H. Lower respiratory tract
I. Cilia
J. Air distributor

_____ 1. Function of respiratory system

_____ 2. Pharynx

_____ 3. Passive transport process responsible for actual exchange of gases

_____ 4. Assists with the movement of mucus towards the pharynx

_____ 5. Barrier between the blood in the capillaries and the air in the alveolus

__B__ 6. Lines the tubes of the respiratory tree

_____ 7. Terminal air sacs

_____ 8. Trachea

_____ 9. Head cold

_____ 10. Homeostatic mechanism

Fill in the blanks.

The organs of the respiratory system are designed to perform two basic functions. They serve as an: (11)__________ __________ and as a (12) __________ __________. In addition to the above, the respiratory system (13) __________, (14) __________, and (15) __________ the air we breathe. Respiratory organs include the (16) __________, (17) __________, (18) __________, (19) __________, (20) __________, and the (21) __________. The respiratory system ends in millions of tiny, thin-walled sacs called (22) __________. (23) __________ of gases takes place in these sacs. Finally, the (24)__________ __________separates the air in the alveoli from the blood in surrounding capillaries and the (25)__________ __________lines most of the air distribution tubes of the respiratory system.

If you have had difficulty with this section, review pages 360-365.

NOSE, PHARYNX, LARYNX

Circle the one that does not *belong.*

26. Nares	Septum	Oropharynx	Conchae
27. Conchae	Frontal	Maxillary	Sphenoidal
28. Oropharynx	Throat	5 inches	Epiglottis
29. Pharyngeal	Adenoids	Uvula	Nasopharynx
30. Middle ear	Tubes	Nasopharynx	Larynx
31. Voice box	Thyroid cartilage	Tonsils	Vocal cords
32. Palatine	Eustachian tube	Tonsils	Oropharynx
33. Pharynx	Epiglottis	Adam's apple	Voice box

Choose the correct term from the options given and write the letter in the answer blank.

(A) Nose (B) Pharynx (C) Larynx

_____ 34. Warms and humidifies air

_____ 35. Air and food pass through here

_____ 36. Sinuses

_____ 37. Conchae

_____ 38. Septum

_____ 39. Tonsils

_____ 40. Middle ear infections

_____ 41. Epiglottis

If you have had difficulty with this section, review pages 365-368.

TRACHEA, BRONCHI, BRONCHIOLES, ALVEOLI, LUNGS, AND PLEURA

Fill in the blanks.

42. The windpipe is more properly referred to as the _______________.
43. _____________ keeps the framework of the trachea almost noncollapsible.
44. _____________ is a major cause of death in the U.S. and includes choking on food and other substances caught in the trachea.
45. The first branch or division of the trachea leading to the lungs is the _____________ _______________.
46. Each alveolar duct ends in several ______________ ___________.
47. The narrow part of each lung, up under the collarbone, is its _______________.
48. The _______________ covers the outer surface of the lungs and lines the inner surface of the rib cage.
49. Inflammation of the lining of the thoracic cavity is ______________.
50. The presence of air in the intrapleural space on one side of the chest is a _____________.

If you have had difficulty with this section, review pages 368-374.

RESPIRATION

True or False

If the statement is true, write "T" in the answer blank. If the statement is false, correct the statement by circling the incorrect term and writing the correct term in the answer blank.

__________________ 51. Diffusion is the process that moves air into and out of the lungs.

__________________ 52. For inspiration to take place, the diaphragm and other respiratory muscles relax.

__________________ 53. Diffusion is a passive process that results in movement up a concentration gradient.

__________________ 54. The exchange of gases that occurs between blood in tissue capillaries and the body cells is external respiration.

__________________ 55. Many pulmonary volumes can be measured as a person breathes into a spirometer.

__________________ 56. Ordinarily we take about 2 pints of air into our lungs.

__________________ 57. The amount of air normally breathed in and out with each breath is called tidal volume.

__________________ 58. The largest amount of air that one can breathe out in one expiration is called residual volume.

__________________ 59. The inspiratory reserve volume is the amount of air that can be forcibly inhaled after a normal inspiration.

If you have had difficulty with this section, review pages 374-380.

Multiple Choice

Circle the correct answer.

60. The term that means the same thing as breathing is:
    A. Gas exchange
    B. Respiration
    C. Inspiration
    D. Expiration
    E. Pulmonary ventilation

61. Carbaminohemoglobin is formed when ______________ binds to hemoglobin.
    A. Oxygen
    B. Amino acids
    C. Carbon dioxide
    D. Nitrogen
    E. None of the above

62. Most of the oxygen transported by the blood is:
    A. Dissolved in white blood cells
    B. Bound to white blood cells
    C. Bound to hemoglobin
    D. Bound to carbaminohemoglobin
    E. None of the above

63. Which of the following would *not* assist inspiration?
    A. Elevation of the ribs
    B. Elevation of the diaphragm
    C. Contraction of the diaphragm
    D. Chest cavity becomes longer from top to bottom

64. A young adult male would have a vital capacity of about __________ ml.
    A. 500
    B. 1200
    C. 3300
    D. 4800
    E. 6200

65. The amount of air that can be forcibly exhaled after expiring the tidal volume is known as the:
    A. Total lung capacity
    B. Vital capacity
    C. Inspiratory reserve volume
    D. Expiratory reserve volume
    E. None of the above

66. Which one of the following is correct?
    A. VC = TV – IRV + ERV
    B. VC = TV + IRV – ERV
    C. VC = TV + IRV x ERV
    D. VC = TV + IRV + ERV
    E. None of the above

If you have had difficulty with this section, review pages 374-380.

REGULATION OF RESPIRATION
RECEPTORS INFLUENCING RESPIRATION
TYPES OF BREATHING

Match the term on the left with the proper selection on the right.

_____	67. Respiratory control centers	A. Difficult breathing
_____	68. Chemoreceptors	B. Located in carotid bodies
_____	69. Pulmonary stretch receptors	C. Slow and shallow respirations
_____	70. Dyspnea	D. Normal respiratory rate
_____	71. Respiratory arrest	E. Located in the medulla
_____	72. Eupnea	F. Failure to resume breathing following a period of apnea
_____	73. Hypoventilation	G. Located throughout pulmonary airways and in the alveoli

If you have had difficulty with this section, review pages 380-385.

UNSCRAMBLE THE WORDS

Take the circled letters, unscramble them, and fill in the statement.

74. **SPUELIRY**

75. **CRNBOSITHI**

76. **SESXPTIAI**

77. **DDNEAOIS**

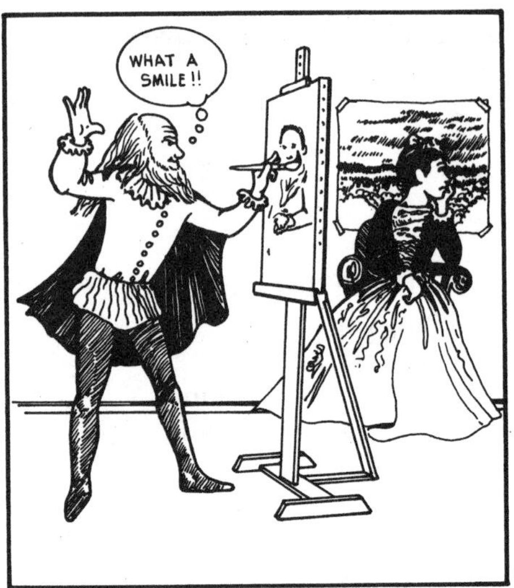

What Mona Lisa was to DaVinci.

78.

APPLYING WHAT YOU KNOW

79. Mr. Gorski is a heavy smoker. Recently he has noticed that when he gets up in the morning, he has a bothersome cough that brings up a large accumulation of mucus. This cough persists for several minutes and then leaves until the next morning. What is an explanation for this problem?

80. Michaela is 5 years old and is a mouth breather. She has had repeated episodes of tonsillitis and the pediatrician has suggested removal of her tonsils and adenoids. He has further suggested that the surgery would probably cure her mouth-breathing problem. Why is this a possibility?

81. WORD FIND

Can you find 14 terms from this chapter in the box of letters? Words may be spelled top to bottom, bottom to top, right to left, left to right, or diagonally.

```
N K S A Q B I L V A D T I X D
O X O O B F I F G I M N R G Y
I G N X W D E E F L B A U T S
T B K Y N H E F O I U T I R P
A T M H E O U T R C C C P V N
L L A E P S I R I Z A A N F E
I P T M I H G T I P R F P C A
T U B O G Q E V A Q O R V N W
N L N G L R J C C R T U P D C
E M U L O V L A U D I S E R E
V O V O T A N G J E D P Z U U
O N K B T C N U U E B O S J S
P A L I I K E U C N O Z K N A
Y R V N S D I O N E D A M F I
H Y O M L O A Z D T Y M N L K
```

Adenoids	Epiglottis	Residual volume
Carotid body	Hypoventilation	Surfactant
Cilia	Inspiration	URI
Diffusion	Oxyhemoglobin	Vital capacity
Dyspnea	Pulmonary	

DID YOU KNOW?

If the alveoli in our lungs were flattened out they would cover a half of a tennis court.

Sinusitis affects 37 million Americans causing difficulty in breathing and chronic headaches.

A person's nose and ears continue to grow throughout his or her life.

RESPIRATORY SYSTEM

Fill in the crossword puzzle.

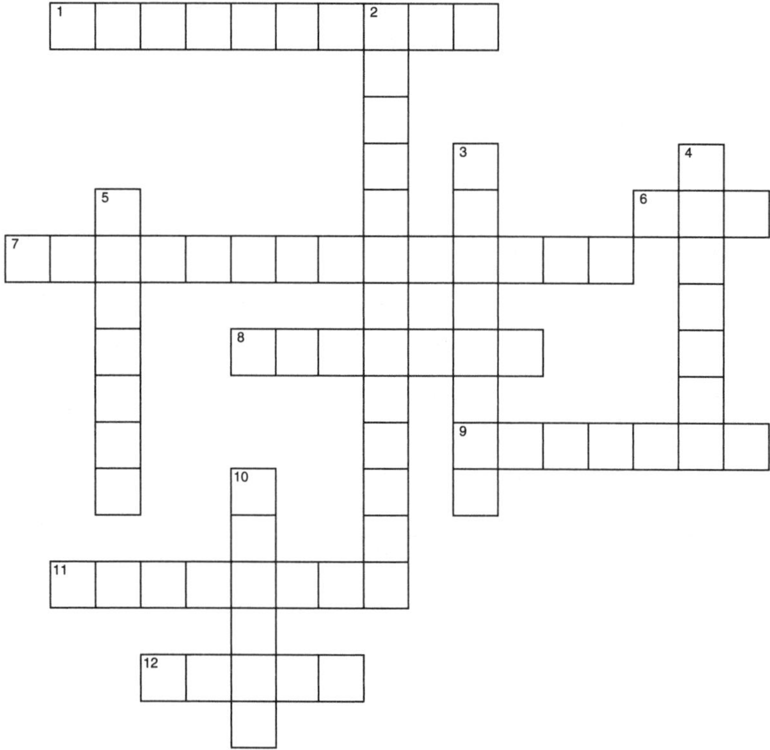

Across

1. Device used to measure the amount of air exchanged in breathing
6. Expiratory reserve volume (abbreviation)
7. Sphenoidal (two words)
8. Terminal air sacs
9. Shelf-like structures that protrude into the nasal cavity
11. Inflammation of pleura
12. Respirations stop

Down

2. Surgical procedure to remove tonsils
3. Doctor who developed lifesaving technique
4. Windpipe
5. Trachea branches into right and left structures
10. Voice box

CHECK YOUR KNOWLEDGE

Multiple Choice

Circle the correct answer.

1. The exchange of gases between the air and blood is made possible by the process of:
   A. Diffusion
   B. Osmosis
   C. Filtration
   D. Pinocytosis

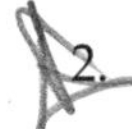

2. Which of the following is *not* a paranasal sinus?
   A. Frontal
   B. Temporal
   C. Maxillary
   D. Sphenoidal

3. The respiratory system serves the body as a(n):
   A. Air distributor
   B. Gas exchanger
   C. Important homeostatic mechanism
   D. All of the above

4. Select the correct pathway that air takes on the way to the lungs.
   A. Primary bronchi, secondary bronchi, alveolar sacs, alveolar ducts
   B. Primary bronchi, secondary bronchi, alveolar sacs, alveoli
   C. Primary bronchi, bronchioles, secondary bronchi, alveolar ducts
   D. Bronchioles, primary bronchi, secondary bronchi, alveoli

5. During expiration:
   A. The thoracic cavity decreases in size
   B. The lungs expand
   C. The diaphragm flattens out and contracts
   D. All of the above

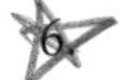

6. The pleura:
   A. Covers the outer surface of the lungs and lines the inner surface of the rib cage
   B. Is an extensive, thin, moist, slippery membrane
   C. Is made up of two membranes known as the parietal pleura and visceral pleura
   D. All of the above

7. The exchange of gases that occurs between blood in tissue capillaries and the body cells is called:
   A. Internal respiration
   B. External respiration
   C. Vital capacity
   D. Inspiratory reserve volume

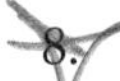

8. Residual volume is the:
   A. Amount of air that can be forcibly inspired over and above a normal inspiration
   B. Amount of air that can be forcibly exhaled after expiring the tidal volume
   C. Air that remains in the lungs after the most forceful expiration
   D. Largest amount of air that we can breathe out in one expiration

9. Eupnea is a term used to describe:
   A. Labored breathing
   B. A temporary stop in breathing
   C. Rapid respirations
   D. A normal respiratory rate

10. The respiratory control centers are located in the:
   A. Cerebrum
   B. Medulla and pons of the brain
   C. Cerebellum
   D. Thalamus

Matching

Select the most correct answer from column B for each statement in column A. (Only one answer is correct.)

Column A	Column B
_____ 11. URI	A. Nostrils
_____ 12. Lower respiratory tract	B. Used to measure air exchange
_____ 13. External nares	C. Carotid and aortic bodies
_____ 14. Voice box	D. C-rings of cartilage
_____ 15. Trachea	E. Head cold
_____ 16. Spirometer	F. Slow, shallow respirations
_____ 17. Chemoreceptors	G. Larynx
_____ 18. Apnea	H. Respiratory arrest
_____ 19. Hypoventilation	I. Chest cold
_____ 20. Apex	J. Lung

SAGITTAL VIEW OF HEAD AND NECK

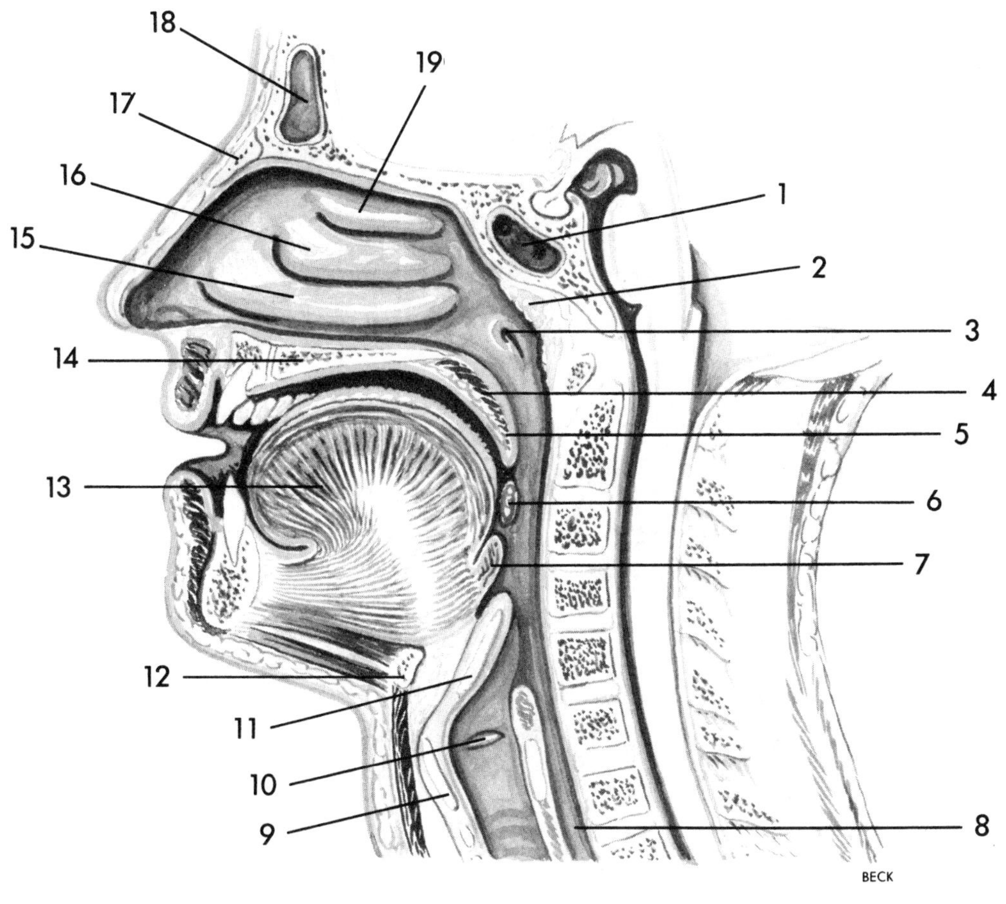

1. ______________________
2. ______________________
3. ______________________
4. ______________________
5. ______________________
6. ______________________
7. ______________________
8. ______________________
9. ______________________
10. ______________________
11. ______________________
12. ______________________
13. ______________________
14. ______________________
15. ______________________
16. ______________________
17. ______________________
18. ______________________
19. ______________________

RESPIRATORY ORGANS

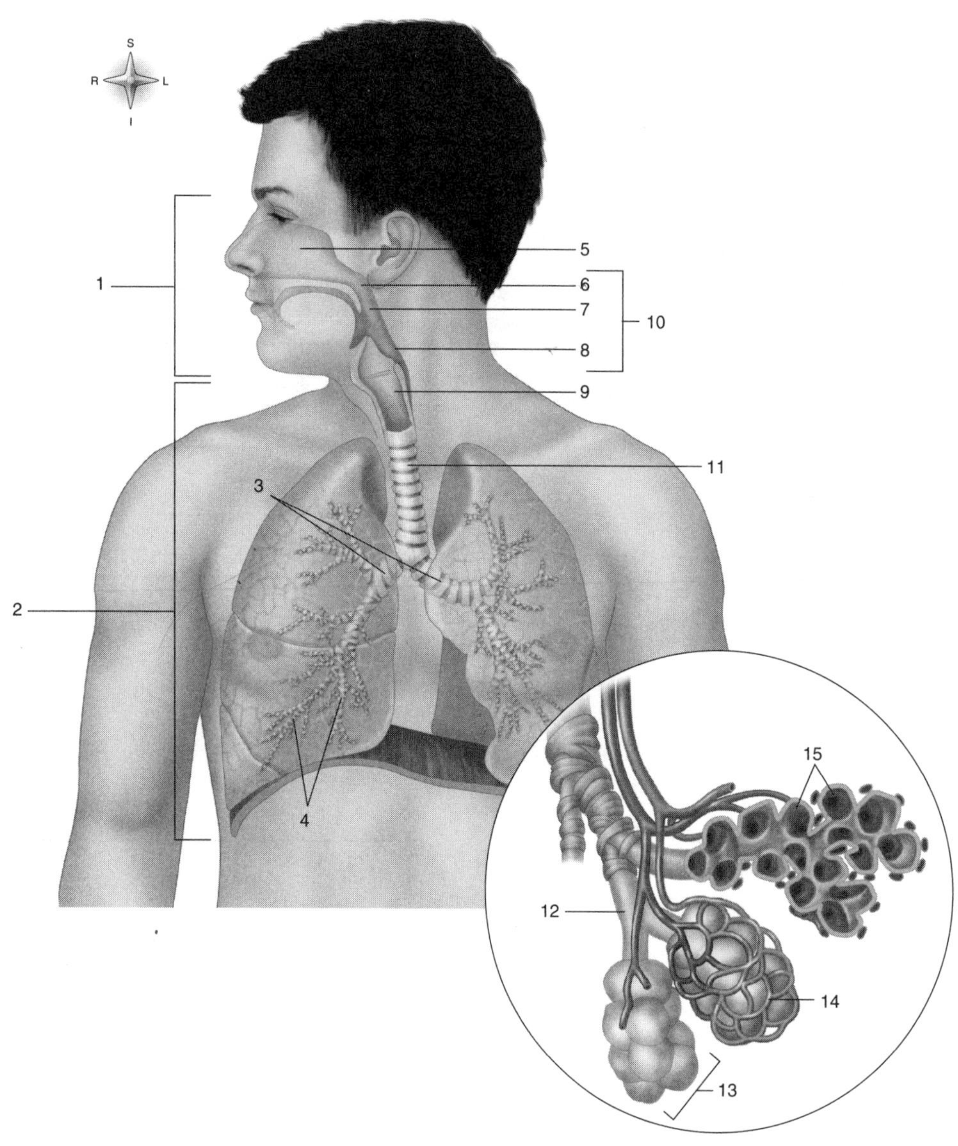

1. Upper digestive tract
2. Lower digestive tract
3. Left and right bronchi
4. bronchioles
5. nasal cavity
6. nasopharynx
7. oropharynx
8. laryngopharynx
9. larynx
10. pharynx
11. trachea
12. alveolar duct
13. alveolar sac
14. capillary
15. alveoli

PULMONARY VENTILATION VOLUMES

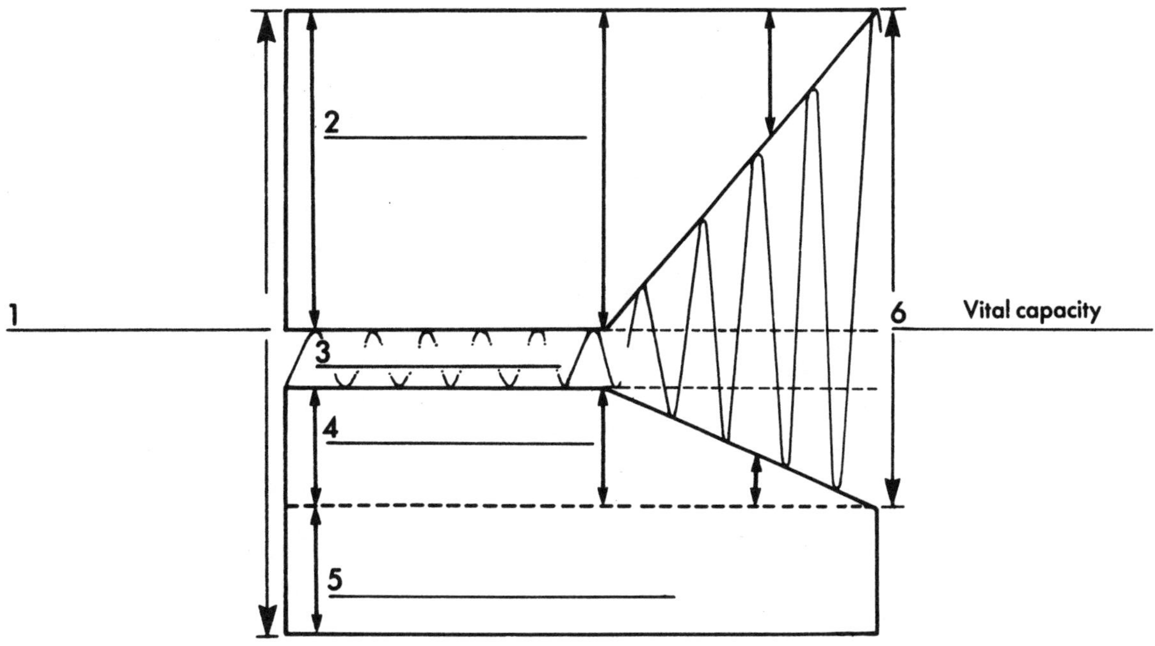

1. ______________________
2. ______________________
3. ______________________
4. ______________________
5. ______________________

CHAPTER 15

The Digestive System

Think of the last meal you ate. Imagine the different shapes, sizes, tastes, and textures that you so recently enjoyed. Think of those items circulating in your bloodstream in those same original shapes and sizes. Impossible? Of course. And because of this impossibility you will begin to understand and marvel at the close relationship of the digestive system to the circulatory system. It is the digestive system that changes our food, both mechanically and chemically, into a form that is acceptable to the blood and the body.

This change begins the moment you take the very first bite. Digestion starts in the mouth, where food is chewed and mixed with saliva. The food then moves down the pharynx and esophagus by peristalsis and enters the stomach. In the stomach it is churned and mixed with gastric juices to become chyme. The chyme goes from the stomach to the duodenum where it is further broken down chemically by intestinal fluids, bile, and pancreatic juice. Those secretions prepare the food for absorption all along the course of the small intestine.

Products that are not absorbed pass on through the entire length of the small intestine (duodenum, jejunum, ileum). From there they enter into the cecum of the large intestine, then the ascending colon, transverse colon, descending colon, sigmoid colon, into the rectum and out the anus.

Products that are used in the cells undergo absorption. Absorption allows newly processed nutrients to pass through the walls of the digestive tract and into the bloodstream to be distributed to the cells.

Your review of this system will help you understand the mechanical and chemical processes necessary to convert food into energy sources and compounds necessary for survival.

TOPICS FOR REVIEW

Before progressing to Chapter 16, you should review the structure and function of all the organs of digestion. You should have an understanding of the process of digestion, both chemical and mechanical, and of the processes of absorption and metabolism.

WALL OF THE DIGESTIVE SYSTEM

Fill in the blanks.

1. The organs of the digestive system form an irregularly shaped tube called the alimentary canal or the ____________ ____________.
2. The churning of food in the stomach is an example of the ____________ breakdown of food.
3. ____________ breakdown occurs when digestive enzymes act on food as it passes through the digestive tract.
4. Waste material resulting from the digestive process is known as ____________.
5. Foods undergo three kinds of processing in the body: ____________, ____________, and ____________.
6. The serosa of the digestive tube is composed of the ____________ ____________ in the abdominal cavity.
7. The digestive tract extends from the ____________ to the ____________.
8. The inside or hollow space within the alimentary canal is called the ____________.
9. The inside layer of the digestive tract is the ____________.
10. The connective tissue layer that lies beneath the lining of the digestive tract is the ____________.
11. The muscularis contracts and moves food through the gastrointestinal tract by a process known as ____________.
12. The outermost covering of the digestive tube is the ____________.
13. The loops of the digestive tract are anchored to the posterior wall of the abdominal cavity by the ____________.

Choose the correct term from the choices given and write the letter in the answer blank.

(A) Main organ (B) Accessory organ

_____ 14. Mouth
_____ 15. Parotids
_____ 16. Liver B
A 17. Stomach
_____ 18. Cecum
A 19. Esophagus
_____ 20. Rectum
A 21. Pharynx
_____ 22. Appendix
_____ 23. Teeth
A 24. Gallbladder
A 25. Pancreas

If you have had difficulty with this section, review pages 390-393.

MOUTH, TEETH, SALIVARY GLANDS

Circle the correct answer.

26. Which one of the following is *not* a part of the roof of the mouth?
    A. Uvula
    B. Palatine bones
    C. Maxillary bones
    D. Soft palate
    E. All of the above are part of the roof of the mouth

27. A thin membrane called the ________ attaches the tongue to the floor of the mouth.
    A. Filiform
    B. Fungiform
    C. Frenulum
    D. Root

28. The first baby tooth, on an average, appears at age:
    A. 2 months
    B. 1 year
    C. 3 months
    D. 1 month
    E. 6 months

29. The portion of the tooth that is covered with enamel is the:
    A. Pulp cavity
    B. Neck
    C. Root
    D. Crown
    E. None of the above

30. The wall of the pulp cavity is surrounded by:
    A. Enamel
    B. Dentin
    C. Cementum
    D. Connective tissue
    E. Blood and lymphatic vessels

31. Which of the following teeth is missing from the deciduous arch?
    A. Central incisor
    B. Canine
    C. Second premolar
    D. First molar
    E. Second molar

32. The permanent central incisor erupts between the ages of ______________.
    A. 9–13
    B. 5–6
    C. 7–10
    D. 7–8
    E. None of the above

33. The third molar appears between the ages of ____________________.
   A. 10–14
   B. 5–8
   C. 11–16
   D. 17–24
   E. None of the above

34. Which one of the following will *not* significantly reduce caries?
   A. Reduction of plaque accumulation on teeth
   B. Fluoride in the water supply
   C. Regular and thorough brushing
   D. Eating a carrot or stick of celery instead of brushing

35. The ducts of the __________________ glands open into the floor of the mouth.
   A. Sublingual
   B. Submandibular
   C. Parotid
   D. Carotid

36. The volume of saliva secreted per day is about:
   A. One-half pint
   B. One pint
   C. One liter
   D. One gallon

37. Mumps are an infection of the:
   A. Parotid gland
   B. Sublingual gland
   C. Submandibular gland
   D. Tonsils

38. Incisors are used during mastication to:
   A. Cut
   B. Piece
   C. Tear
   D. Grind

39. Another name for the third molar is:
   A. Central incisor
   B. Wisdom tooth
   C. Canine
   D. Lateral incisor

40. After food has been chewed, it is formed into a small rounded mass called a:
   A. Moat
   B. Chyme
   C. Bolus
   D. Protease

If you have had difficulty with this section, review pages 393-398.

-4

PHARYNX, ESOPHAGUS, STOMACH

Fill in the blanks.

The (41) ________________ is a tubelike structure that functions as part of both respiratory and digestive systems. It connects the mouth with the (42) ____________________. The esophagus serves as a passageway for movement of food from the pharynx to the (43) ________________. Food enters the stomach by passing through the muscular (44) ________________ ________________ at the end of the esophagus. Contraction of the stomach mixes the food thoroughly with the gastric juices and breaks it down into a semisolid mixture called (45) ____________________.

The three divisions of the stomach are the (46) ________________, (47) ________________, and (48) ________________.

Food is held in the stomach by the (49) ________________ ________________ muscle long enough for partial digestion to occur. After food has been in the stomach for approximately 3 hours, the chyme will enter the (50) ________________ ____________________.

Match the term with the correct definition.

A. Esophagus
B. Chyme
C. Peristalsis
D. Rugae
E. Triple therapy
F. Greater curvature
G. Hiatal hernia
H. Pepcid
I. Acid indigestion
J. Lesser curvature

_____ 51. Stomach folds

_____ 52. Upper right border of stomach

_____ 53. Condition that may result in backward movement or reflux of stomach contents into the lower portion of the esophagus

_____ 54. 10-inch passageway

_____ 55. Drug used to treat GERD

_____ 56. Semisolid mixture of stomach contents

_____ 57. Muscle contractions of the digestive system

_____ 58. Used to heal ulcers and prevent recurrences

_____ 59. Heartburn

_____ 60. Lower left border of stomach

If you have had difficulty with this section, review pages 398-403.

SMALL INTESTINE, LIVER AND GALLBLADDER, PANCREAS

Circle the correct answer.

61. Which one is *not* part of the small intestine?
    A. Jejunum
    B. Ileum
    C. Cecum
    D. Duodenum

62. Which one of the following structures does *not* increase the surface area of the intestine for absorption?
    A. Plicae
    B. Rugae
    C. Microvilli
    D. Villi

63. The union of the cystic duct and hepatic duct form the:
    A. Common bile duct
    B. Major duodenal papilla
    C. Minor duodenal papilla
    D. Pancreatic duct

64. Obstruction of the ____________________ will lead to jaundice.
    A. Hepatic duct
    B. Pancreatic duct
    C. Cystic duct
    D. None of the above

65. Each villus in the intestine contains a lymphatic vessel or ____________________ that serves to absorb lipid or fat materials from the chyme.
    A. Plica
    B. Lacteal
    C. Villa
    D. Microvilli

66. The middle third of the duodenum contains the:
    A. Islets
    B. Fundus
    C. Body
    D. Rugae
    E. Major duodenal papilla

67. Most gastric and duodenal ulcers result from infection with the bacterium:
    A. Biaxin
    B. Metronidazole
    C. Prilosec
    D. *Helicobacter pylori*

68. The liver is an:
    A. Enzyme
    B. Endocrine organ
    C. Endocrine gland
    D. Exocrine gland

69. Fats in chyme stimulate the secretion of the hormone:
    A. Lipase
    B. Cholecystokinin
    C. Protease
    D. Amylase

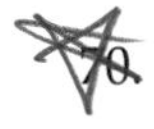
70. The largest gland in the body is the:
   A. Pituitary
   B. Thyroid
   C. Liver
   D. Thymus

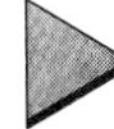
If you have had difficulty with this section, review pages 403-406.

LARGE INTESTINE, APPENDIX, PERITONEUM

If the statement is true, write "T" in the answer blank. If the statement is false, correct the statement by circling the incorrect term and writing the correct term in the answer blank.

______________ 71. Bacteria in the large intestine are responsible for the synthesis of vitamin E needed for normal blood clotting.

______________ 72. Villi in the large intestine absorb salts and water.

______________ 73. If waste products pass rapidly through the large intestine, constipation results.

______________ 74. The ileocecal valve opens into the sigmoid colon.

______________ 75. The splenic flexure is the bend between the ascending colon and the transverse colon.

______________ 76. The splenic colon is the S-shaped segment that terminates in the rectum.

______________ 77. The appendix serves no important digestive function in humans.

______________ 78. For patients with suspected appendicitis, a physician will often evaluate the appendix by a digital rectal examination.

______________ 79. The visceral layer of the peritoneum lines the abdominal cavity.

______________ 80. The greater omentum is shaped like a fan and serves to anchor the small intestine to the posterior abdominal wall.

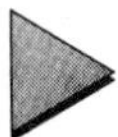
If you have had difficulty with this section, review pages 406-412.

DIGESTION, ABSORPTION, METABOLISM

Circle the correct answer.

81. Which one of the following substances does *not* contain any enzymes?
   A. Saliva
   B. Bile
   C. Gastric juice
   D. Pancreatic juice
   E. Intestinal juice

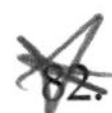
82. Which one of the following is a simple sugar?
   A. Maltose
   B. Sucrose
   C. Lactose
   D. Glucose
   E. Starch

83. Cane sugar is the same as:
    A. Maltose
    B. Lactose
    C. Sucrose
    D. Glucose
    E. None of the above

84. Most of the digestion of carbohydrates takes place in the:
    A. Mouth
    B. Stomach
    C. Small intestine
    D. Large intestine

85. Fats are broken down into:
    A. Amino acids
    B. Simple sugars
    C. Fatty acids
    D. Disaccharides

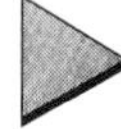 *If you have had difficulty with this section, review pages 412-416.*

CHEMICAL DIGESTION

86. *Fill in the blank areas on the chart below.*

DIGESTIVE JUICES AND ENZYMES	SUBSTANCE DIGESTED (OR HYDROLYZED)	RESULTING PRODUCT
Saliva		
1. Amylase	1.	1. Maltose (disaccharide)
Gastric Juice		
2. Protease (pepsin) plus hydrochloric acid	2. Proteins	2.
Pancreatic Juice		
3. Proteases (e.g., trypsin)	3. Proteins (intact or partially digested)	3.
4. Lipases	4.	4. Fatty acids, monoglycerides, and glycerol
5. Amylase	5.	5. Maltose
Intestinal Enzymes		
6. Peptidases	6.	6. Amino acids
7.	7. Sucrose	7. Glucose and fructose
8. Lactase	8.	8. Glucose and galactose (simple sugars)
9. Maltase	9. Maltose	9.

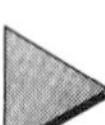 *If you have had difficulty with this section, review page 414, Table 15-2.*

UNSCRAMBLE THE WORDS

Take the circled letters, unscramble them, and fill in the statement.

87. **S L B O U**

88. **E Y C H M**

89. **L L A A P P I**

90. **P M E R T E U I O N**

What the groom gave his bride after the wedding.

91.

APPLYING WHAT YOU KNOW

92. Mr. Amato was a successful businessman, but he worked too hard and was always under great stress. His doctor cautioned him that if he did not alter his style of living he would be subject to hyperacidity. What could be the resulting condition of hyperacidity?

93. Baby Shearer has been regurgitating his bottle feeding at every meal. The milk is curdled, but does not appear to be digested. He has become dehydrated, and so his mother is taking him to the pediatrician. What is a possible diagnosis from your textbook reading?

94. Mr. Attanas has gained a great deal of weight suddenly. He also noticed that he was sluggish and always tired. What test might his physician order for him and for what reason?

95. WORD FIND

Can you find the 22 terms from the chapter in the box of letters? Words may be spelled top to bottom, bottom to top, right to left, left to right, or diagonally.

```
X M E T A B O L I S M X X W
R S D P E R I S T A L S I S
E V A M N O I T S E G I D R
E D E E U O Q T W Q O H N Q
Q Z H S R N I N T F E C E S
D H R E C C I T K C J A P E
Q W R N A T N V P Y R M P C
O C A T N R B A P R H O A I
U Y I E O W T A P A O T W D
B O D R L N P B F Q J S V N
N T S Y F I S L U M E E B U
W G J A L U V U N R N W O A
Q S N L X D U O D E N U M J
H C A V I T Y M U C O S A D
Y E A A P H V W S V C Q J C
```

Absorption	Emulsify	Mucosa
Appendix	Feces	Pancreas
Cavity	Fundus	Papillae
Crown	Heartburn	Peristalsis
Dentin	Jaundice	Stomach
Diarrhea	Mastication	Uvula
Digestion	Mesentery	
Duodenum	Metabolism	

DID YOU KNOW?

The liver performs over 500 functions and produces over 1000 enzymes to handle the chemical conversions necessary for survival.

The human stomach lining replaces itself every 3 days.

Even if the stomach, the spleen, 75% of the liver, 80% of the intestines, one kidney, one lung, and virtually every organ from the pelvic and groin area are removed, the human body can still survive!

DIGESTIVE SYSTEM

Fill in the crossword puzzle.

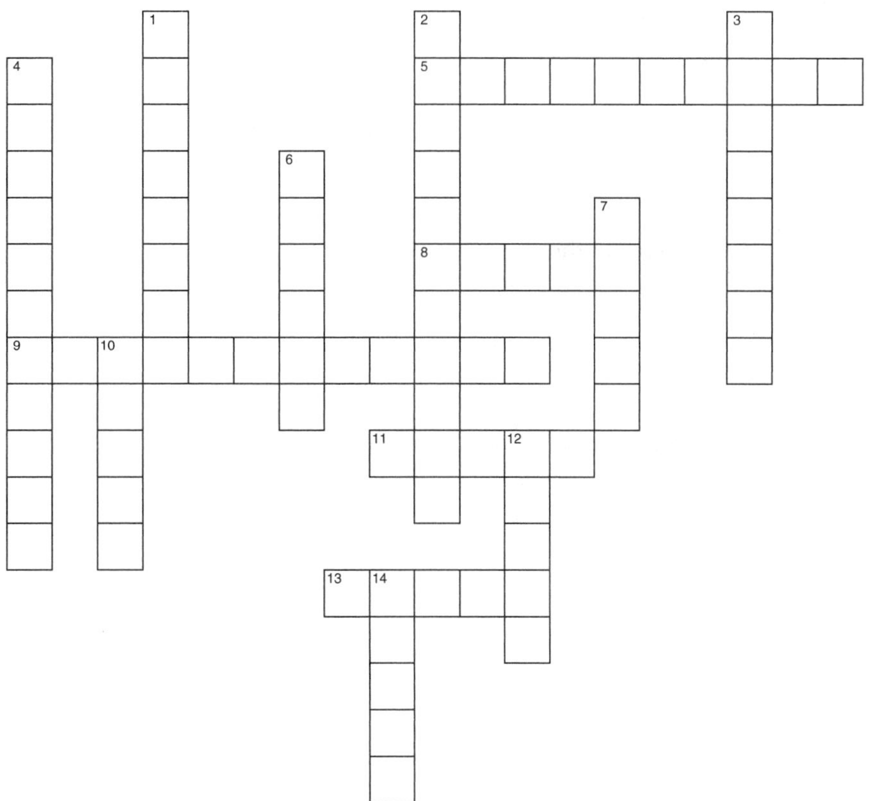

Across

5. Digested food moves from intestine to blood
8. Semisolid mixture
9. Inflammation of the appendix
11. Rounded mass of food
13. Stomach folds

Down

1. Yellowish skin discoloration
2. Process of chewing
3. Fluid stools
4. Movement of food through digestive tract
6. Vomitus
7. Waste product of digestion
10. Intestinal folds
12. Open wound in digestive area acted on by acid juices
14. Prevents food from entering nasal cavities

CHECK YOUR KNOWLEDGE

Multiple Choice

Circle the correct answer.

1. The principal structure of the digestive system is an irregular tube, open at both ends, and is called the:
   A. Alimentary canal
   B. Oral cavity
   C. Colon
   D. Esophagus

2. Which of the following is *not* a layer of the digestive tract?
   A. Mucosa
   B. Muscularis
   C. Lumen
   D. Serosa

3. Which of the following is *not* a main organ of the digestive system?
   A. Liver
   B. Stomach
   C. Cecum
   D. Colon

4. Which of the following classification of teeth have a cutting function during mastication?
   A. Canines
   B. Incisors
   C. Premolars
   D. Molars

5. Which of the following is an accurate description of the salivary glands?
   A. There are four pairs of salivary glands.
   B. Salivary amylase begins the chemical digestion of carbohydrates.
   C. They are located within the digestive tube.
   D. The submandibular glands are the ones involved when people have the mumps.

6. The act of swallowing moves a mass of food called a _______ from the mouth to the stomach.
   A. Dentin
   B. Bolus
   C. Chyme
   D. Frenulum

7. Stomach muscle contractions result in:
   A. Rugae
   B. Peristalsis
   C. Plicae
   D. None of the above

8. The stomach sphincter that keeps food from reentering the esophagus when the stomach contracts is known as the:
   A. Hiatal
   B. Pyloric
   C. Cardiac
   D. Fundus

9. Most of the chemical digestion occurs in the:
   A. Stomach
   B. Liver
   C. Duodenum
   D. Jejunum

10. The pancreas:
    A. Is an exocrine gland
    B. Contains enzymes that digest proteins and fats only
    C. Contains an acid substance that elevates the pH of the gastric juice
    D. None of the above

COMPLETION

Complete the following statements.

11. Undigested and unabsorbed food materials enter the large intestine after passing through a sphincterlike structure called the ____________________ ____________________.

12. The subdivisions of the large intestine in the order in which food material or feces pass through them are: cecum, ascending colon, transverse colon, descending colon, ____________________ ____________________, rectum, and anal canal.

13. The vermiform appendix is directly attached to the ____________________.

14. The ____________________ is an extension between the parietal and visceral layers of the peritoneum and is shaped like a giant, pleated fan.

15. Chewing, swallowing, peristalsis, and defecation are the main processes of ________________ ________________.

16. The end products of carbohydrate digestion are ____________________.

17. The end products of protein digestion are____________________.

18. The end products of fat digestion are ____________________ and ____________________.

19. The process by which molecules of amino acids, glucose, fatty acids, and glycerol go from the inside of the intestines into the circulating fluids of the body is known as ____________________.

20. Three intestinal enzymes____________________, ____________________, and ____________________digest disaccharides by changing them into monosaccharides.

-3

DIGESTIVE ORGANS

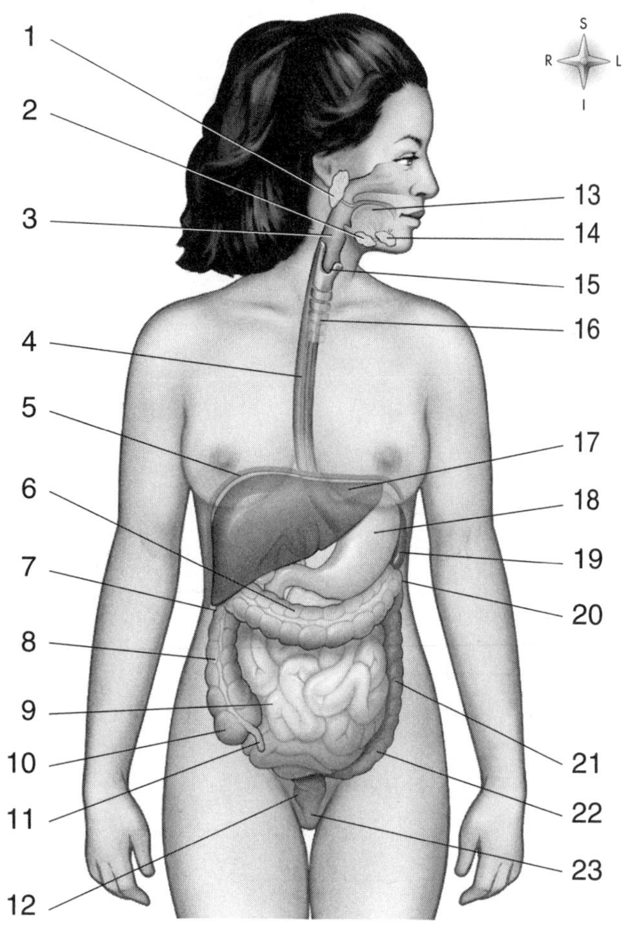

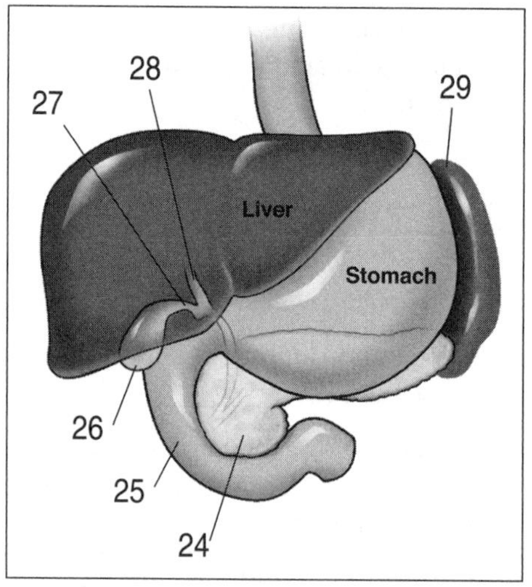

1.	______________________	16.	______________________
2.	______________________	17.	______________________
3.	______________________	18.	______________________
4.	______________________	19.	______________________
5.	______________________	20.	______________________
6.	______________________	21.	______________________
7.	______________________	22.	______________________
8.	______________________	23.	______________________
9.	______________________	24.	______________________
10.	______________________	25.	______________________
11.	______________________	26.	______________________
12.	______________________	27.	______________________
13.	______________________	28.	______________________
14.	______________________	29.	______________________
15.	______________________		

TOOTH

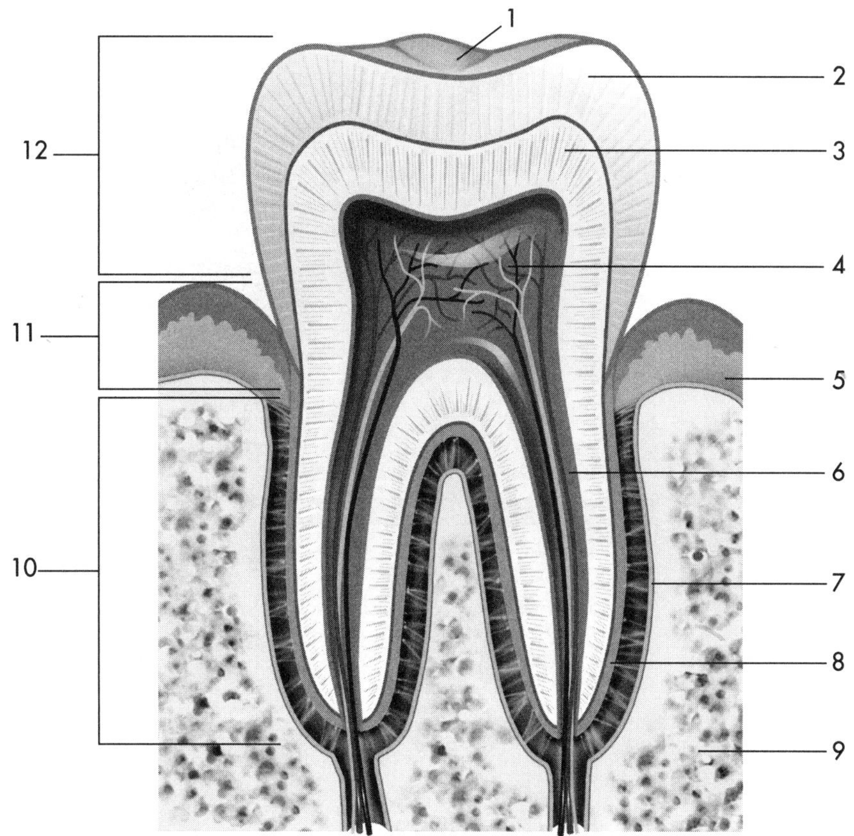

1. ______________________
2. ______________________
3. ______________________
4. ______________________
5. ______________________
6. ______________________
7. ______________________
8. ______________________
9. ______________________
10. ______________________
11. ______________________
12. ______________________

THE SALIVARY GLANDS

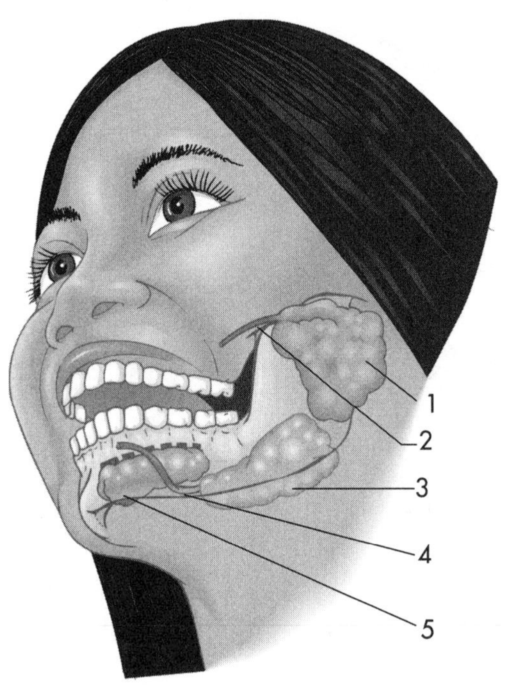

1. ______________________
2. ______________________
3. ______________________
4. ______________________
5. ______________________

STOMACH

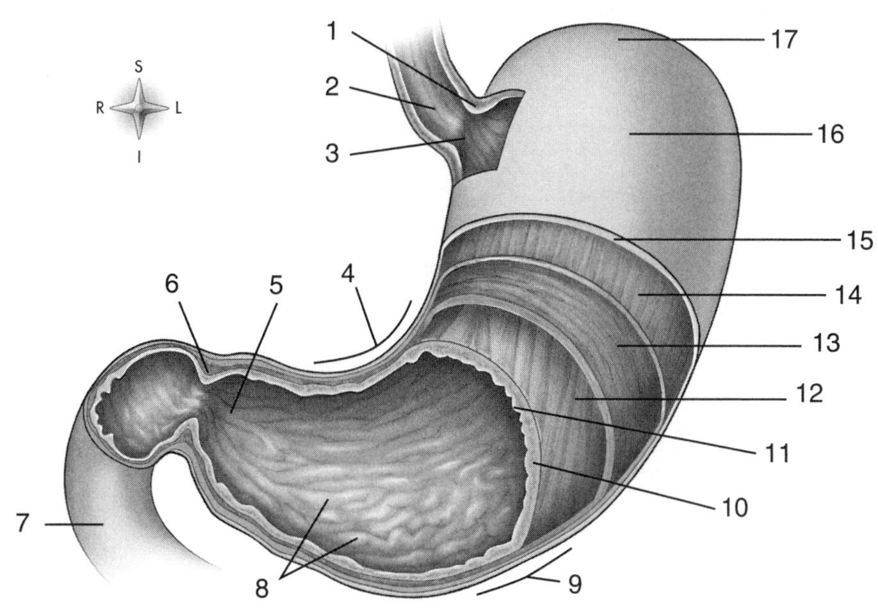

1. ______________________
2. ______________________
3. ______________________
4. ______________________
5. ______________________
6. ______________________
7. ______________________
8. ______________________
9. ______________________
10. ______________________
11. ______________________
12. ______________________
13. ______________________
14. ______________________
15. ______________________
16. ______________________
17. ______________________

GALLBLADDER AND BILE DUCTS

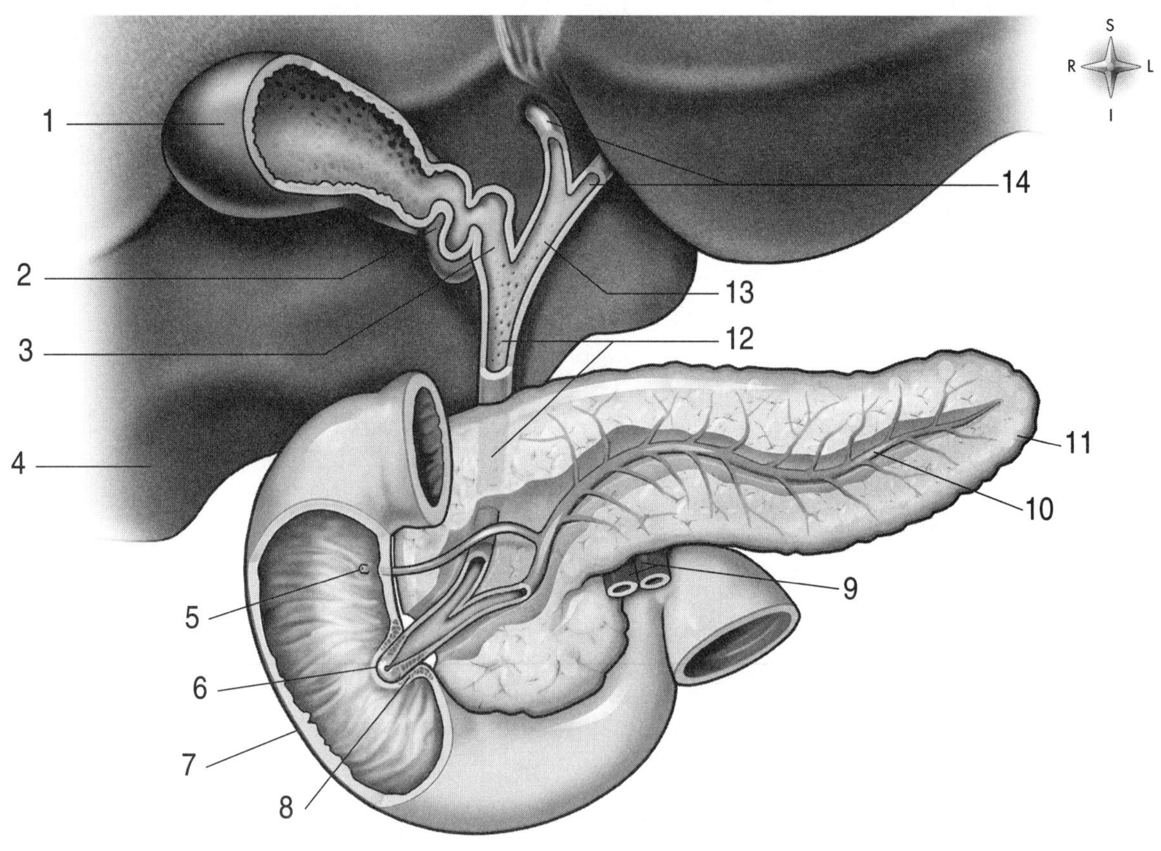

1. ______________________
2. ______________________
3. ______________________
4. ______________________
5. ______________________
6. ______________________
7. ______________________
8. ______________________
9. ______________________
10. ______________________
11. ______________________
12. ______________________
13. ______________________
14. ______________________

THE SMALL INTESTINE

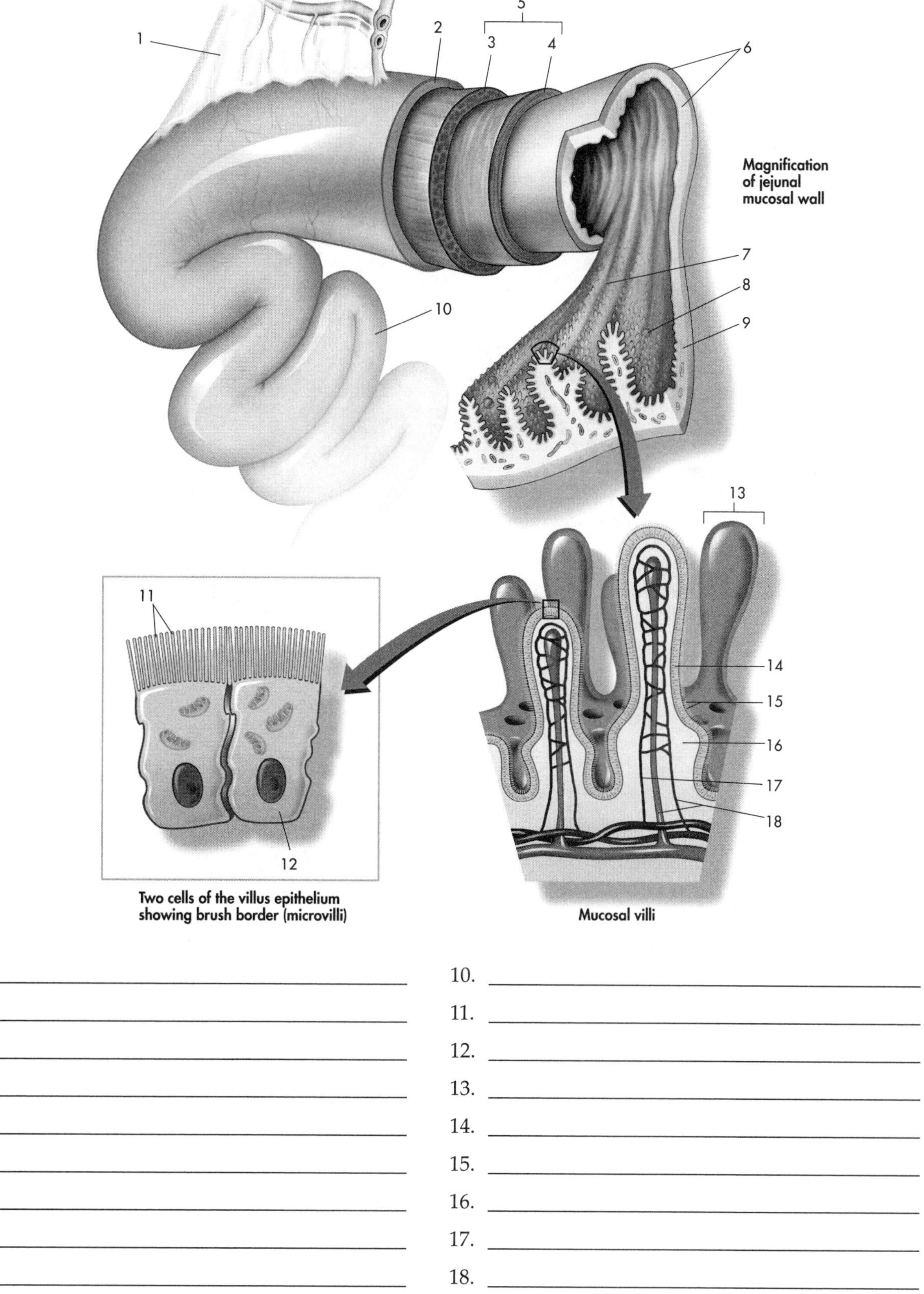

1. ______________________
2. ______________________
3. ______________________
4. ______________________
5. ______________________
6. ______________________
7. ______________________
8. ______________________
9. ______________________
10. ______________________
11. ______________________
12. ______________________
13. ______________________
14. ______________________
15. ______________________
16. ______________________
17. ______________________
18. ______________________

THE LARGE INTESTINE

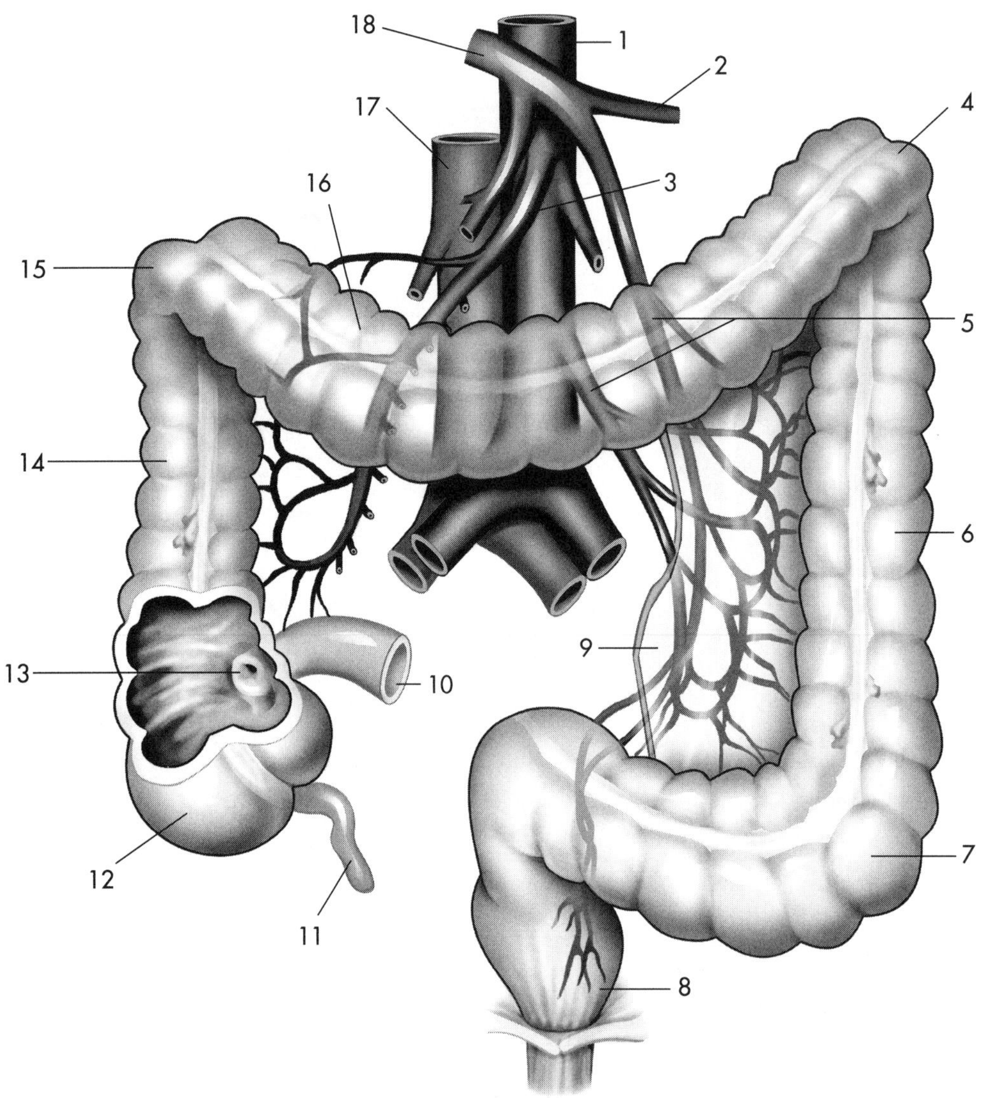

1. ______________________
2. ______________________
3. ______________________
4. ______________________
5. ______________________
6. ______________________
7. ______________________
8. ______________________
9. ______________________
10. ______________________
11. ______________________
12. ______________________
13. ______________________
14. ______________________
15. ______________________
16. ______________________
17. ______________________
18. ______________________

CHAPTER 16

Nutrition and Metabolism

Most of us love to eat, but do the foods we enjoy provide us with the basic food types necessary for good nutrition? The body, a finely tuned machine, requires a balance of carbohydrates, fats, proteins, vitamins, and minerals to function properly. These nutrients must be digested, absorbed, and circulated to cells constantly to accommodate the numerous activities that occur throughout the body. The use the body makes of foods once these processes are completed is called "metabolism."

The liver plays a major role in the metabolism of food. It helps maintain a normal blood glucose level, removes toxins from the blood, processes blood immediately after it leaves the gastrointestinal tract, and initiates the first steps of protein and fat metabolism.

This chapter also discusses basal metabolic rate (BMR). The BMR is the rate at which food is catabolized under basal conditions. This test and the measurement of the amount of protein-bound iodine (PBI) are indirect measures of thyroid gland functioning. The total metabolic rate (TMR) is the amount of energy, expressed in calories, used by the body each day.

Finally, maintaining a constant body temperature is a function of the hypothalamus and a challenge for the metabolic factors of the body. Review of this chapter is necessary to provide you with an understanding of the "fuel" or nutrition necessary to maintain your complex homeostatic machine—the body.

TOPICS FOR REVIEW

Before progressing to Chapter 17, you should be able to define and contrast catabolism and anabolism. Your review should include the metabolic roles of carbohydrates, fats, proteins, vitamins, and minerals. Your study should conclude with an understanding of the basal metabolic rate and physiological mechanisms that regulate body temperature.

THE ROLE OF THE LIVER

Fill in the blanks.

The liver plays an important role in the mechanical digestion of lipids because it secretes (1) ___________________. It also produces two of the plasma proteins that play an essential role in blood clotting: (2) _______________ and (3) _______________. Additionally, liver cells store several substances, notably vitamins A and D and (4) _____________. Finally, the liver is assisted by a unique structural feature of the blood vessels that supply it. This arrangement, known as the (5) _________ _________ __________, allows toxins to be removed from the bloodstream before nutrients are distributed throughout the body.

If you have had difficulty with this section, review pages 422-424.

NUTRIENT METABOLISM

Match the term on the left with the proper selection of the right.

(A) Carbohydrates (B) Fats (C) Proteins (D) Vitamins (E) Minerals

_____ 6. Used if cells have inadequate amounts of glucose to catabolize
_____ 7. Preferred energy food
_____ 8. Amino acids
_____ 9. Fat soluble
_____ 10. Required for nerve conduction
_____ 11. Glycolysis
_____ 12. Inorganic elements found naturally in the earth
_____ 13. Pyruvic acid

Circle the one that does not *belong.*

14. Glycolysis	Citric acid cycle	ATP	Bile
15. Adipose	Amino acids	Triglycerides	Glycerol
16. A	D	M	K
17. Iron	Proteins	Amino acids	Essential
18. Hydrocortisone	Insulin	Growth hormone	Epinephrine
19. Sodium	Calcium	Zinc	Folic acid
20. Thiamine	Niacin	Ascorbic acid	Riboflavin

If you have had difficulty with this section, review pages 424-428.

METABOLIC RATES, BODY TEMPERATURE

Circle the correct answer.

21. The rate at which food is catabolized under basal conditions is the:
    A. TMR
    B. PBI
    C. BMR
    D. ATP

22. The total amount of energy used by the body per day is the:
    A. TMR
    B. PBI
    C. BMR
    D. ATP

23. Over ___________ of the energy released from food molecules during catabolism is converted to heat rather than being transferred to ATP.
    A. 20%
    B. 40%
    C. 60%
    D. 80%

24. Maintaining thermoregulation is a function of the:
    A. Thalamus
    B. Hypothalamus
    C. Thyroid
    D. Parathyroids

25. Transfer of heat energy to the skin and then to the external environment is known as:
    A. Radiation
    B. Conduction
    C. Convection
    D. Evaporation

26. A flow of heat waves away from the blood is known as:
    A. Radiation
    B. Conduction
    C. Convection
    D. Evaporation

27. A transfer of heat energy to air that is continually flowing away from the skin is known as:
    A. Radiation
    B. Conduction
    C. Convection
    D. Evaporation

28. Heat absorbed by the process of water vaporization is called:
    A. Radiation
    B. Conduction
    C. Convection
    D. Evaporation

29. A(n) ________________ is the amount of energy needed to raise the temperature of 1 gram of water 1° C.
    A. Calorie
    B. Kilocalorie
    C. ATP
    D. BMR

If you have had difficulty with this section, review pages 428-433.

UNSCRAMBLE THE WORDS

Take the circled letters, unscramble them, and fill in the statement.

30. **L R I E V**

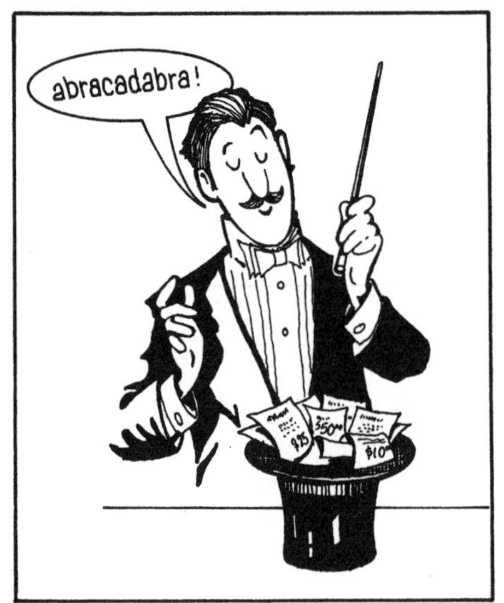

31. **T A O B A L I C M S**

32. **O M N I A**

33. **Y P U R C V I**

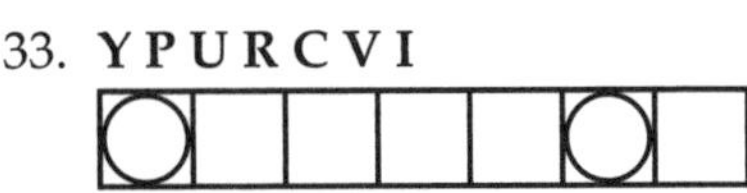

How the magician paid his bills.

34.

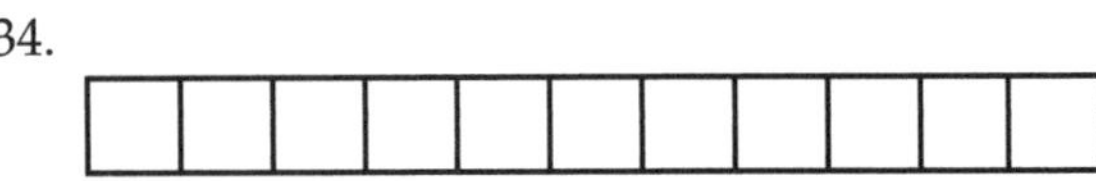

APPLYING WHAT YOU KNOW

35. Dr. Culp was concerned about Deborrah. Her daily food intake provided fewer calories than her TMR. If this trend continues, what will be the result? If it continues over a long period of time, what eating disorder might Deborrah develop?

36. Mrs. Bishop was experiencing fatigue and a blood test revealed that she was slightly anemic. What mineral will her doctor most likely prescribe? What dietary sources might you suggest that she emphasize in her daily intake?

37. Mrs. Hosmer was training daily for an upcoming marathon. Three days before the 26-mile event, she suddenly quit her daily routine of jogging and switched to a diet high in carbohydrates. Why did Mrs. Hosmer suddenly switch her routine of training?

38. WORD FIND

Can you find 18 terms from this chapter in the box of letters? Words may be spelled top to bottom, bottom to top, right to left, left to right, or diagonally.

```
C C C B W E F F L J V G G S
A T N L W E U O Z I E L I B
R K K P Z F R I T P O Y K L
B Q M I N E R A L S J C C P
O S S N C X M I D B D O W P
H S I Y O I T X H I N L S N
Y E L N N I K W W D S Y N S
D G O S O W T I U E H S C N
R M B Y T I W C Z N N I A A
A R A Q W A T B E I G S J M
T E T F N I F A E V E W T Y
E V A P O R A T I O N D T E
S I C N E S O P I D A O F E
H L Y K I R E B V P A H C J
I W E E P A D F T E A R G G
```

ATP	Conduction	Liver
Adipose	Convection	Minerals
BMR	Evaporation	Proteins
Bile	Fats	Radiation
Carbohydrates	Glycerol	TMR
Catabolism	Glycolysis	Vitamins

DID YOU KNOW?

Twenty-five years ago, 3%–5% of Americans were deficient in vitamin C. Today, about 15% don't get the amount they need for optimum health.

The human body has enough fat to produce 7 bars of soap.

Forty to fifty percent of body heat can be lost through the head (no hat) as a result of its extensive circulatory network.

NUTRITION/METABOLISM

Fill in the crossword puzzle.

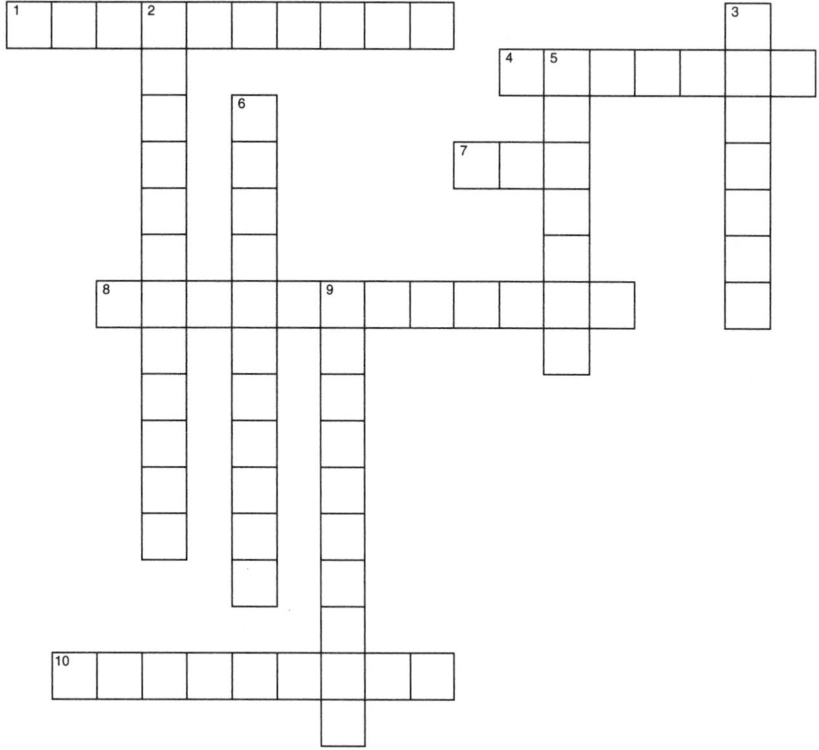

Across

1. Breaks food molecules down releasing stored energy
4. Amount of energy needed to raise the temperature of one gram of water 1° Celsius
7. Rate of metabolism when a person is lying down, but awake (abbreviation)
8. A series of reactions that join glucose molecules together to form glycogen
10. Builds food molecules into complex substances

Down

2. Occurs when food molecules enter cells and undergo many chemical changes there
3. Organic molecule needed in small quantities for normal metabolism throughout the body
5. Oxygen-using
6. A unit of measure for heat, also known as a large calorie
9. Takes place in the cytoplasm of a cell and changes glucose to pyruvic acid

CHECK YOUR KNOWLEDGE

Multiple Choice

Circle the correct answer.

1. Metabolism is a term that refers to the:
   A. Nutrients that we eat
   B. Use of foods
   C. Building blocks
   D. None of the above

2. Glycolysis changes glucose into:
   A. Pyruvic acid
   B. Carbon dioxide
   C. ATP
   D. None of the above

3. An anaerobic process:
   A. Is an oxygen-using process
   B. Is an oxygen-storing process
   C. Uses no oxygen
   D. Both A and B

4. The amount of nutrients in the blood:
   A. Changes significantly when we exercise
   B. Changes significantly when we go without food for many hours
   C. Does not change very much and remains relatively constant
   D. Both A and B

5. Which of the following hormones lowers blood glucose levels?
   A. Growth hormone
   B. Insulin
   C. Hydrocortisone
   D. Epinephrine

6. Fats not needed for catabolism are anabolized to form:
   A. Nonessential amino acids
   B. Triglycerides
   C. Glycogen
   D. ATP

7. Essential amino acids:
   A. Must be in the diet
   B. Can be made by the body
   C. Make up the majority of the 20 amino acids
   D. All of the above

8. A good source of iron in the diet is:
   A. Meat
   B. Dairy products
   C. Seafood
   D. Fruits

9. The flow of heat waves away from the blood is known as:
   A. Conduction
   B. Radiation
   C. Convection
   D. Evaporation

10. The liver:
    A. Plays an important role in the mechanical digestion of lipids because it secretes bile
    B. Detoxifies various poisonous substances such as bacterial products and certain drugs
    C. Synthesizes several kinds of protein compounds
    D. All of the above

Completion

Complete the following statements.

11. The preferred energy food of the body is ____________________.
12. An anaerobic process is ____________________.
13. An aerobic process is the ____________ ____________ ____________.
14. A deficiency of ____________ may result in a goiter.
15. The rate at which food is catabolized under basal conditions is known as the ____________ ____________ ____________.
16. The total amount of energy used by the body per day is the ____________ ____________ ____________.
17. Maintaining homeostasis of temperature is the function of the ____________________.
18. Night blindness may occur as a result of a deficiency of vitamin ____________.
19. A good source of folic acid in the diet is ____________________.
20. Four fat-soluble vitamins that can be stored in the liver for later use are: ____________, ____________, ____________, and ____________.

CHAPTER 17

The Urinary System

Living produces wastes. Wherever people live or work or play, wastes accumulate. To keep these areas healthy, there must be a method—such as a sanitation department—of disposing of these wastes.

Wastes accumulate in your body also. The conversion of food and gases into substances and energy necessary for survival results in waste products. A large percentage of these wastes is removed by the urinary system.

Two vital organs, the kidneys, cleanse the blood of the many waste products that are continually produced as a result of the metabolism of food in the body cells. They eliminate these wastes in the form of urine.

Urine formation is the result of three processes: filtration, reabsorption, and secretion. These processes occur in successive portions of the microscopic units of the kidneys known as nephrons. The amount of urine produced by the nephrons is controlled primarily by the hormones ADH and aldosterone.

After urine is produced it is drained from the renal pelvis by the ureters to flow into the bladder. The bladder then stores the urine until it is voided through the urethra.

If waste products are allowed to accumulate in the body they soon become poisonous, a condition called uremia. A knowledge of the urinary system is necessary to understand how the body rids itself of waste and avoids toxicity.

TOPICS FOR REVIEW

Before progressing to Chapter 18 you should have an understanding of the structure and function of the organs of the urinary system. Your review should include knowledge of the nephron and its role in urine production. Your study should conclude with a review of the three main processes involved in urine production and the mechanisms that control urine volume.

KIDNEYS

Multiple Choice

Circle the correct answer.

1. The outermost portion of the kidney is known as the:
   A. Medulla
   B. Papilla
   C. Pelvis
   D. Pyramid
   E. Cortex

2. The saclike structure that surrounds the glomerulus is the:
   A. Renal pelvis
   B. Calyx
   C. Bowman's capsule
   D. Cortex
   E. None of the above

3. The renal corpuscle is made up of the:
   A. Bowman's capsule and proximal convoluted tubule
   B. Glomerulus and proximal convoluted tubule
   C. Bowman's capsule and the distal convoluted tubule
   D. Glomerulus and the distal convoluted tubule
   E. Bowman's capsule and the glomerulus

4. Which of the following functions is *not* performed by the kidneys?
   A. Maintenance of homeostasis
   B. Removal of wastes from the blood
   C. Production of ADH
   D. Removal of electrolytes from the blood

5. ____________ percent of the glomerular filtrate is reabsorbed.
   A. Twenty
   B. Forty
   C. Seventy-five
   D. Eighty-five
   E. Ninety-nine

6. The glomerular filtration rate is ________________ ml per minute.
   A. 1.25
   B. 12.5
   C. 125.0
   D. 1250.0
   E. None of the above

7. Glucose is reabsorbed in the:
   A. Loop of Henle
   B. Proximal convoluted tubule
   C. Distal convoluted tubule
   D. Glomerulus
   E. None of the above

8. Reabsorption does *not* occur in the:
   A. Loop of Henle
   B. Proximal convoluted tubule
   C. Distal convoluted tubule
   D. Collecting tubules
   E. Calyx

9. The greater the amount of salt intake, the:
   A. Less salt excreted in the urine
   B. More salt is reabsorbed
   C. More salt excreted in the urine
   D. None of the above

10. Which one of the following substances is secreted by diffusion?
    A. Sodium ions
    B. Certain drugs
    C. Ammonia
    D. Hydrogen ions
    E. Potassium ions

11. Which of the following statements about ADH is *not* true?
    A. It is stored by the pituitary gland.
    B. It makes the collecting tubules less permeable to water.
    C. It makes the distal convoluted tubules more permeable.
    D. It is produced by the hypothalamus.

12. Which of the following statements about aldosterone is *not* true?
    A. It is secreted by the adrenal cortex.
    B. It is a water-retaining hormone.
    C. It is a salt-retaining hormone.
    D. All of the above are correct.

If you have had difficulty with this section, review pages 438-448.

Matching

Choose the correct term and write the letter in the space next to the appropriate definition below.

A. Medulla
B. Cortex
C. Pyramids
D. Papilla
E. Pelvis
F. Calyx
G. Nephrons
H. Uremia
I. Proteinuria
J. Bowman's capsule
K. Glomerulus
L. Loop of Henle
M. CAPD
N. Glycosuria

_____ 13. Functioning unit of urinary system

_____ 14. Abnormally large amounts of plasma proteins in the urine

_____ 15. Uremic poisoning

_____ 16. Outer part of kidney

_____ 17. Together with Bowman's capsule forms renal corpuscle

_____ 18. Division of the renal pelvis

_____ 19. Cup-shaped top of a nephron

_____ 20. Innermost end of a pyramid

_____ 21. Extension of proximal tubule

_____ 22. Triangular-shaped divisions of the medulla of the kidney

_____ 23. Used in the treatment of renal failure

_____ 24. Inner portion of kidney

If you have had difficulty with this section, review pages 441-450.

URETERS, URINARY BLADDER, URETHRA

Indicate which organ is identified by the following descriptions by writing the appropriate letter in the answer blank.

(A) Ureters (B) Bladder (C) Urethra

_____ 25. Rugae

_____ 26. Lowermost part of urinary tract

_____ 27. Lining membrane richly supplied with sensory nerve endings

_____ 28. Lies behind pubic symphysis

_____ 29. Dual function in male

_____ 30. 1½ inches long in female

_____ 31. Drains renal pelvis

_____ 32. Surrounded by prostate in male

_____ 33. Elastic fibers and involuntary muscle fibers

_____ 34. 10–12 inches long

_____ 35. Trigone

Fill in the blanks.

36. ________________ ________________ is the description of the pain caused by the passage of a kidney stone.
37. The urinary tract is lined with ________________ ________________.
38. Another name for kidney stones is ________________ ________________.
39. A technique that uses ________________ to pulverize stones, thus avoiding surgery, is being used to treat kidney stones.
40. Older people generally have a lower overall lean body mass, and therefore, a ________________ production of waste products that must be excreted from the body.
41. The ________________ ________________ is the basinlike upper end of the ureter located inside the kidney.
42. In the male, the urethra serves as a passageway for both urine and ________________.
43. The external opening of the urethra is the ________________ ________________.

If you have had difficulty with this section, review pages 448-451.

MICTURITION

Fill in the blanks.

The terms (44) ____________, (45) ____________ and (46) ____________ all refer to the passage of urine from the body or the emptying of the bladder. The sphincters guard the bladder. The (47)____________ ____________ sphincter is located at the bladder (48) ____________ and is involuntary. The external urethral sphincter circles the (49) ____________ and is under (50) ____________ control.

As the bladder fills, nervous impulses are transmitted to the spinal cord and an (51) ____________ ____________ is initiated. Urine then enters the (52) ____________ to be eliminated.

Urinary (53) ____________ is a condition in which no urine is voided. Urinary (54) ____________ is when the kidneys do not produce any urine, but the bladder retains its ability to empty itself. Complete destruction or transection of the sacral cord produces an (55) ____________ ____________.

If you have had difficulty with this section, review pages 451-452.

UNSCRAMBLE THE WORDS

Take the circled letters, unscramble them, and fill in the statement.

56. **AYXLC**

57. **GVNOIDI**

58. **ALPALIP**

59. **SGULLOUMRE**

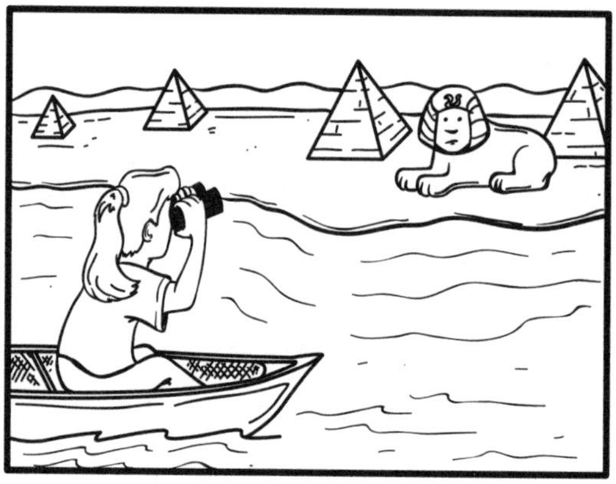

What Betty saw while cruising down the Nile.

60.

APPLYING WHAT YOU KNOW

61. John suffered from low levels of ADH. What primary urinary symptom would he notice?

62. Bud was in a diving accident and his spinal cord was severed. He was paralyzed from the waist down and as a result was incontinent. His physician was concerned about the continuous residual urine build-up. What was the reason for concern?

63. Caryl had a prolonged surgical procedure and experienced problems with urinary retention postoperatively. A urinary catheter was inserted into her bladder for the elimination of urine. Several days later Caryl developed cystitis. What might be a possible cause?

64. WORD FIND

Can you find 18 terms from the chapter in the box of letters? Words may be spelled top to bottom, bottom to top, right to left, left to right, or diagonally.

```
H N O I T I R U T C I M N M Y
V E Q N G A L L I P A P S E S
T P M C O L D U J Y S I N D D
L H G O X I O W C G V D I U J
C R F N D B T M T L I M B K L
P O O T X I C A E K A P X L D
Q N U I E G A P R R T C W A O
B J R N T T L L Y T U Y G D M
S D E E R G Y P Y V L L P H Z
I H T N O U X W D S X I U J G
M X E C C Y S T I T I S F S Q
J O R E D D A L B U E S G B S
Y I S E B V L L B H V Q L U L
```

ADH	Filtration	Micturition
Bladder	Glomerulus	Nephron
Calculi	Hemodialysis	Papilla
Calyx	Incontinence	Pelvis
Cortex	Kidney	Pyramids
Cystitis	Medulla	Ureters

DID YOU KNOW?

If the tubules in a kidney were stretched out and untangled, there would be 70 miles of them.

While examining urine, German chemist Hennig Brand discovered phosphorus.

URINARY SYSTEM

Fill in the crossword puzzle.

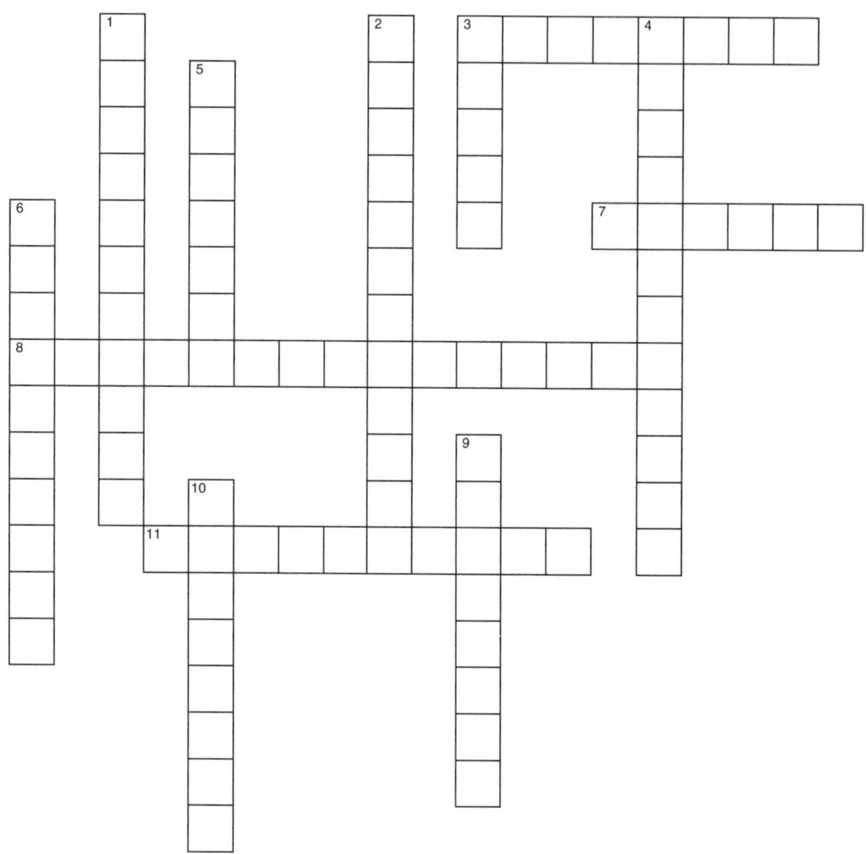

Across

3. Bladder infection
7. Absence of urine
8. Passage of a tube into the bladder to withdraw urine
11. Network of blood capillaries tucked into Bowman's capsule

Down

1. Urination
2. Ultrasound generator used to break up kidney stones
3. Division of the renal pelvis
4. Voiding involuntarily
5. Area on posterior bladder wall free of rugae
6. Glucose in the urine
9. Large amount of urine
10. Scanty urine

CHECK YOUR KNOWLEDGE

Multiple Choice

Circle the correct answer.

1. Which of the following is *not* true of the kidneys?
   A. The right kidney is lower than the left.
   B. They are retroperitoneal.
   C. The rate of blood flow through the kidneys is among the highest in the body.
   D. All of the above are true.

2. Bowman's capsule and the glomerulus make up the:
   A. Renal tubule
   B. Renal corpuscle
   C. Loop of Henle
   D. Collecting tubule

3. The kidneys serve the body by:
   A. Maintaining homeostasis
   B. Excreting toxins and waste products containing nitrogen
   C. Regulating the proper balance between body water content and salt
   D. All of the above

4. Urine formation begins with:
   A. Glomerular filtration
   B. The proximal convoluted tubule
   C. The distal convoluted tubule
   D. The loop of Henle

5. A well-known sign of diabetes mellitus is:
   A. Proteinuria
   B. Oliguria
   C. Glycosuria
   D. Anuria

6. A lithotriptor is used for:
   A. Diabetes mellitus
   B. Incontinence
   C. Renal calculi
   D. Oliguria

7. Aldosterone:
   A. Assists in controlling the kidney tubules' excretion of salt
   B. Simulates the tubules to reabsorb sodium salts at a faster rate
   C. Decreases tubular water reabsorption
   D. Is a salt- and water-losing hormone

8. Control of urine volume is maintained primarily by the:
   A. Bowman's capsule
   B. Loop of Henle
   C. ADH from the posterior pituitary gland
   D. Kidney tubule

9. Which is *not* a part of the kidney?
   A. Cortex
   B. Trigone
   C. Medulla
   D. Pyramids

10. Which of the following is *not* a primary process in urine formation?
   A. Active transport
   B. Filtration
   C. Reabsorption
   D. Secretion

Matching

Select the most correct answer from column B for each statement in column A. (Only one answer is correct.)

	Column A	Column B
_____	11. Uremia	A. Urinary bladder infection
_____	12. Nephrons	B. Triangular divisions of medulla of kidney
_____	13. Renal tubule	C. Microscopic units of kidney
_____	14. Juxtaglomerular apparatus	D. Blood pressure regulation
_____	15. Secretion	E. Uremic poisoning
_____	16. CAPD	F. Loop of Henle
_____	17. Cystitis	G. Relaxation of internal sphincter
_____	18. Emptying reflex	H. Renal failure
_____	19. Calyces	I. Divisions of renal pelvis
_____	20. Pyramids	J. Hydrogen and potassium ions

URINARY SYSTEM

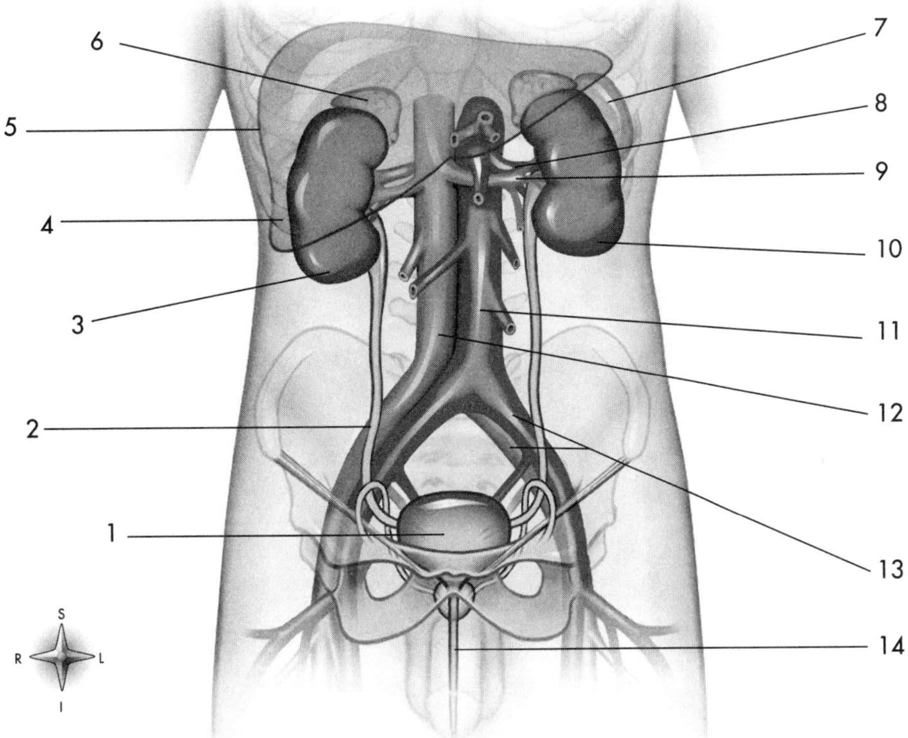

1. ______________________
2. ______________________
3. ______________________
4. ______________________
5. ______________________
6. ______________________
7. ______________________
8. ______________________
9. ______________________
10. ______________________
11. ______________________
12. ______________________
13. ______________________
14. ______________________

KIDNEY

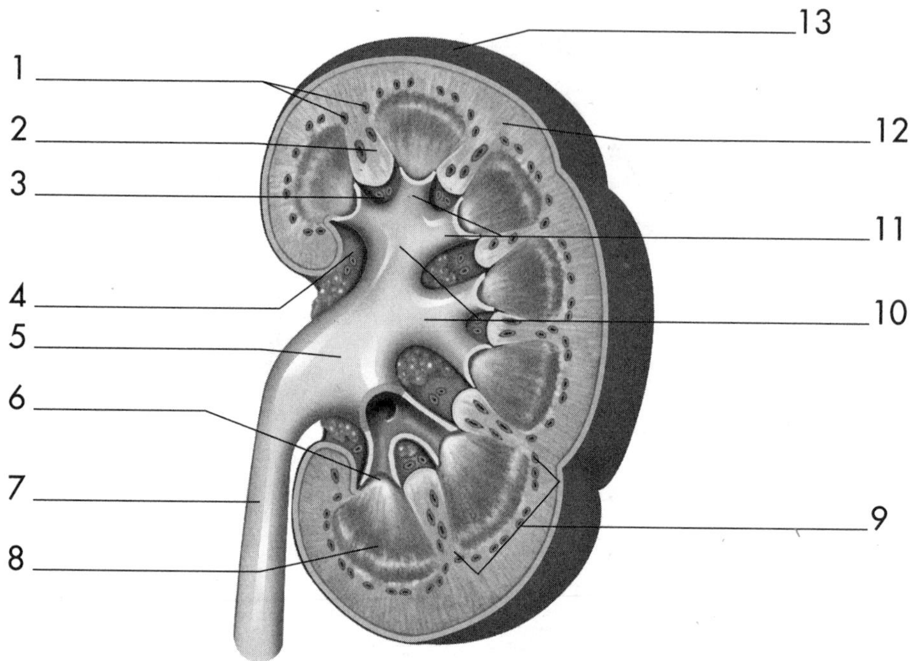

1. Interlobular arteries
2. Renal column
3. Renal Sinus
4. Hilum
5. Renal pelvis
6. Renal papilla of pyramid
7. Ureter
8. Medulla
9. medullary pyramid
10. major calyces
11. minor calyces
12. cortex
13. capsule

NEPHRON

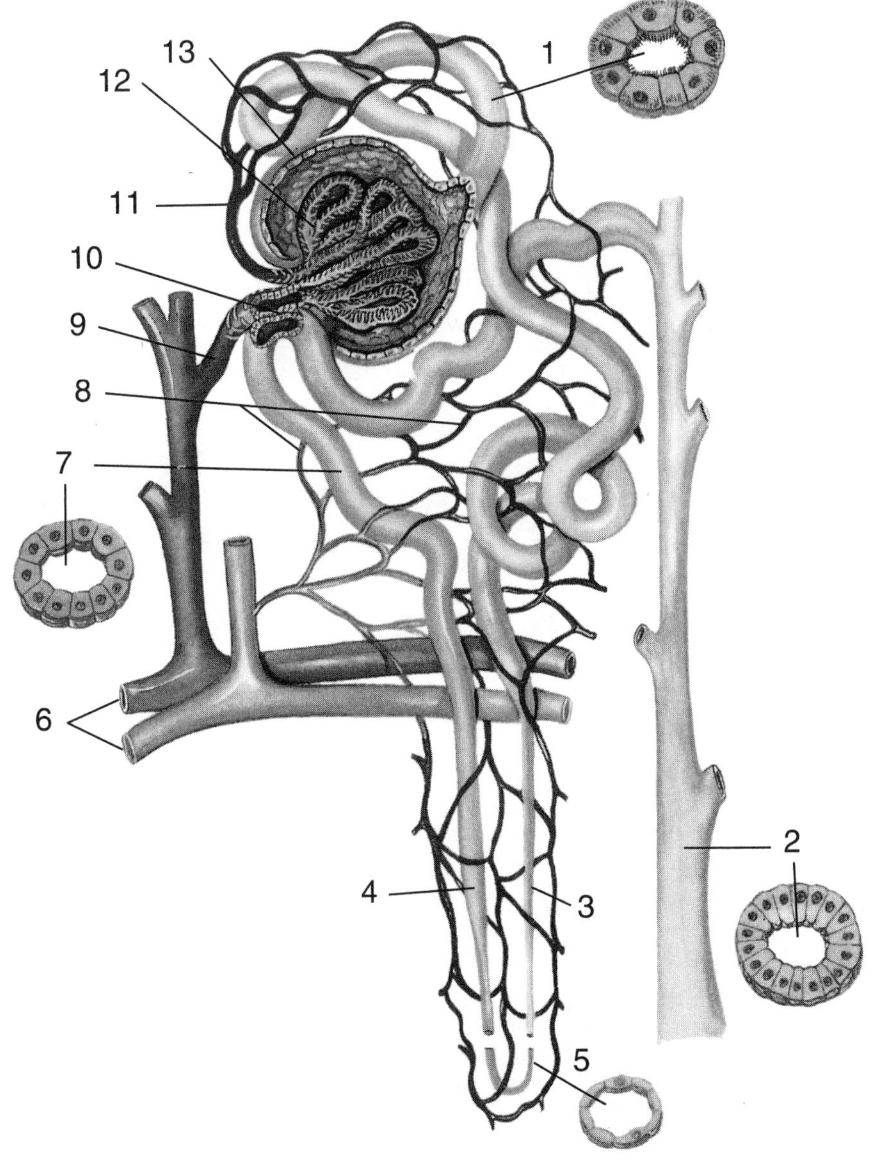

1. ______________________
2. ______________________
3. ______________________
4. ______________________
5. ______________________
6. ______________________
7. ______________________
8. ______________________
9. ______________________
10. ______________________
11. ______________________
12. ______________________
13. ______________________

CHAPTER 18

Fluid and Electrolyte Balance

In the very first chapter of the your text, you learned that survival depends on the body's ability to maintain or restore homeostasis. Specifically, homeostasis means that the body fluids remain constant within very narrow limits. These fluids are classified as either intracellular fluid (ICF) or extracellular fluid (ECF). As the names imply, intracellular fluid lies within the cells and extracellular fluid is located outside the cells. A balance between these two fluids is maintained by certain body mechanisms: (a) the adjustment of fluid output to fluid intake under normal circumstances; (b) the concentration of electrolytes in the extracellular fluid; (c) the capillary blood pressure; and (d) the concentration of proteins in the blood.

Comprehension of how these mechanisms maintain and restore fluid balance is necessary for an understanding of the complexities of homeostasis and its relationship to the survival of the individual.

TOPICS FOR REVIEW

Before progressing to Chapter 19, you should review the types of body fluids and their subdivisions. Your study should include the mechanisms that maintain fluid balance and the nature and importance of electrolytes in body fluids. You should be able to give examples of common fluid imbalances and have an understanding of the role of fluid and electrolyte balance in the maintenance of homeostasis.

BODY FLUIDS

Circle the correct answer.

1. The largest volume of water by far lies (inside or outside) cells.
2. Interstitial fluid is (intracellular or extracellular).
3. Plasma is (intracellular or extracellular).
4. Obese people have a (lower or higher) water content per pound of body weight than thin people.
5. Infants have (more or less) water in comparison to body weight than adults of either sex.
6. There is a rapid (increase or decline) in the proportion of body water to body weight during the first 10 years of life.
7. The female body contains slightly (more or less) water per pound of weight.
8. In general, as age increases, the amount of water per pound of body weight (increases or decreases).
9. Excluding adipose tissue, approximately (55% or 85%) of body weight is water.
10. The term (fluid balance or fluid compartments) means the volumes of ICF, IF, plasma, and the total volume of water in the body all remain relatively constant.

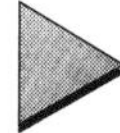
If you have had difficulty with this section, review pages 458-462.

MECHANISMS THAT MAINTAIN FLUID BALANCE

Multiple Choice

Circle the correct answer.

11. Which one of the following is a positively charged ion?
    A. Sodium
    B. Chloride
    C. Phosphate
    D. Bicarbonate

12. Which one of the following is a negatively charged ion?
    A. Sodium
    B. Potassium
    C. Calcium
    D. Chloride

13. The most abundant electrolytes in the blood plasma are:
    A. NaCl
    B. KMg
    C. HCO_3
    D. HPO_4
    E. $CaPO_4$

14. If the blood sodium concentration increases, then blood volume will:
    A. Increase
    B. Decrease
    C. Remain the same
    D. None of the above

15. The smallest amount of water comes from:
   A. Water in foods that are eaten
   B. Ingested liquids
   C. Water formed from catabolism
   D. None of the above

16. The greatest amount of water lost from the body is from the:
   A. Lungs
   B. Skin, by diffusion
   C. Skin, by sweat
   D. Feces
   E. Kidneys

17. Which one of the following is *not* a major factor that influences extracellular and intracellular fluid volumes?
   A. The concentration of electrolytes in the extracellular fluid
   B. The capillary blood pressure
   C. The concentration of proteins in blood
   D. All of the above are major factors

18. The type of fluid output that changes the most is:
   A. Water loss in the feces
   B. Water loss across the skin
   C. Water loss via the lungs
   D. Water loss in the urine
   E. None of the above

19. The chief regulators of sodium within the body is (are) the:
   A. Lungs
   B. Sweat glands
   C. Kidneys
   D. Large intestine
   E. None of the above

20. Which of the following is *not* correct?
   A. Fluid output must equal fluid intake.
   B. ADH controls salt reabsorption in the kidney.
   C. Water follows sodium.
   D. Renal tubule regulation of salt and water is the most important factor in determining urine volume.

21. Diuretics work on all of the following *except*:
   A. Proximal tubule
   B. Loop of Henle
   C. Distal tubule
   D. Collecting ducts
   E. Diuretics work on all of the above

22. Of all the sodium-containing secretions, the one with the largest volume is:
   A. Saliva
   B. Gastric secretions
   C. Bile
   D. Pancreatic juice
   E. Intestinal secretions

23. The higher the capillary blood pressure, the ____________ the amount of interstitial fluid.
    A. Smaller
    B. Larger
    C. There is no relationship between capillary blood pressure and volume of interstitial fluid

24. An increase in capillary blood pressure will lead to ____________ in blood volume.
    A. An increase
    B. A decrease
    C. No change
    D. None of the above

25. Which one of the fluid compartments varies the most in volume?
    A. Intracellular
    B. Interstitial
    C. Extracellular
    D. Plasma

26. Which one of the following will *not* cause edema?
    A. Retention of electrolytes in the extracellular fluid
    B. Increase in capillary blood pressure
    C. Burns
    D. Decrease in plasma proteins
    E. All of the above may cause edema

True or False

If the statement is true, write "T" in the answer blank. If the statement is false, correct the statement by circling the incorrect term and writing the correct term in the answer blank.

____________ 27. The three sources of fluid intake are the liquids we drink, the foods we eat, and the water formed by the anabolism of foods.

____________ 28. The body maintains fluid balance mainly by changing the volume of urine excreted to match changes in the volume of fluid intake.

____________ 29. Some output of fluid will occur as long as life continues.

____________ 30. Glucose is an example of an electrolyte.

____________ 31. Where sodium goes, water soon follows.

____________ 32. Excess aldosterone leads to hypovolemia.

____________ 33. Diuretics have their effect on glomerular function.

____________ 34. Typical daily intake and output totals should be approximately 1200 ml.

____________ 35. Bile is a sodium-containing internal secretion.

____________ 36. The average daily diet contains about 500 mEq of sodium.

If you have had difficulty with this section, review pages 462-468.

FLUID IMBALANCES

Fill in the blanks.

(37)_______________ is the fluid imbalance seen most often. In this condition, interstitial fluid volume (38) ________________ first, but eventually, if treatment has not been given, intracellular fluid and plasma volumes (39) __________________. (40) __________________ can also occur, but is much less common.

Giving (41) ___________ ________ too rapidly or in too large amounts can put too heavy a burden on the (42) ________________.

If you have had difficulty with this section, review pages 468-470.

APPLYING WHAT YOU KNOW

43. Mrs. Titus was asked to keep an accurate record of her fluid intake and output. She was concerned because the two did not balance. What is a possible explanation for this?

44. Nurse Briker was caring for a patient who was receiving diuretics. What special nursing implications should be followed for patients on this therapy?

45. WORD FIND

Can you find the 12 terms from this chapter in the box of letters? Words may be spelled top to bottom, bottom to top, right to left, left to right, or diagonally.

```
S T V H O M E O S T A S I S H
I E D E M A S Q A L P U E G L
M M L U F L U I D O Y O I S L
W S B E A E C O L D P N I E R
L I T A C V S H Q O C E H B C
L L X J L T E A W Y B V Q Q O
I O O P E A R U C T C A A R I
N B H R X S N O I I P R T C N
S A O X M G J C L N J T B A H
I N X X D V U D E Y K N Y O C
E A A J Q D I U R E T I C S X
I F C J A M P V E N B E Y F W
V F K T Q X R M D D S I V O T
E T T Z N T R P X I M L J F I
S W Y A P V Q N S K T K W B P
```

Aldosterone	Edema	Imbalance
Anabolism	Electrolyte	Intravenous
Catabolism	Fluid	Ions
Diuretics	Homeostasis	Kidney

DID YOU KNOW?

The best fluid replacement drink is 1/4 teaspoon of table salt to one quart of water.

If all of the water were drained from the body of an average 160-pound man, the body would weigh 64 pounds.

FLUID/ELECTROLYTES

Fill in the crossword puzzle.

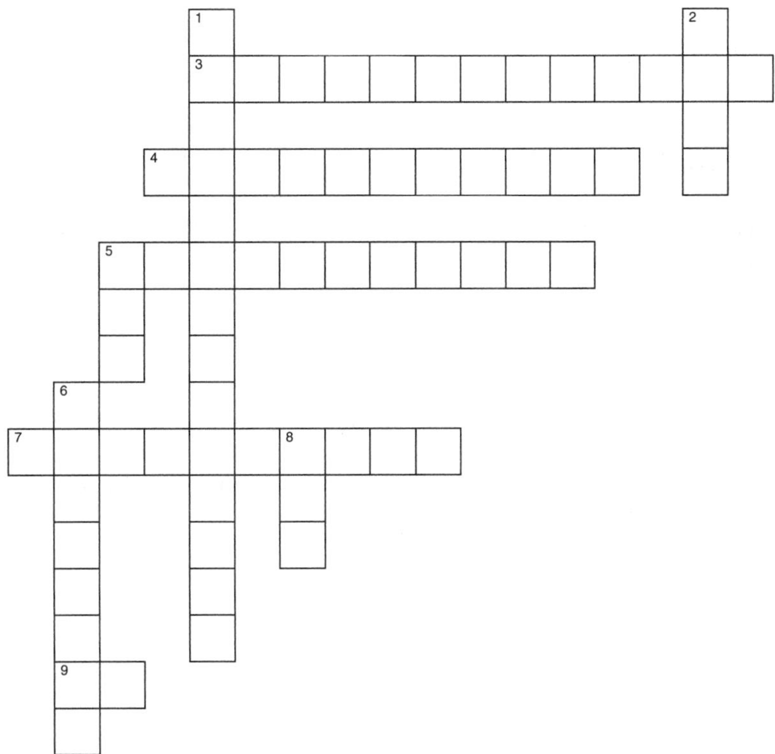

Across

3. Result of rapidly given intravenous fluids
4. Result of large loss of body fluids
5. Compound that dissociates in solution into ions
7. To break up
9. A subdivision of extracellular fluid (abbreviation)

Down

1. Organic substance that doesn't dissociate in solution
2. Dissociated particles of an electrolyte that carry an electrical charge
5. Fluid outside cells (abbreviation)
6. "Causing urine"
8. Fluid inside cells (abbreviation)

CHECK YOUR KNOWLEDGE

Multiple Choice

Circle the correct answer.

1. Which of the following have the most water compared to body weight?
   A. Infants
   B. Females
   C. Males
   D. All of the above have the same percentage of water to body weight

2. Which of the following acts as a mechanism for controlling plasma, IF, and ICF volumes?
   A. The concentration of electrolytes in ECF
   B. The capillary blood pressure
   C. The concentration of proteins in blood
   D. All of the above

3. Which of the following statements is true regarding maintenance of fluid homeostasis?
   A. The type of fluid output that changes most is urine volume.
   B. Renal tubule regulation of salt and water is the most important factor in determining urine volume.
   C. The presence of sodium causes water to move.
   D. All of the above are true.

4. Which of the following is *not* a normal portal of exit for water from the body?
   A. Diffusion
   B. Lungs
   C. Water formed by catabolism
   D. Intestines

5. The fluid imbalance that is seen most often is:
   A. Dehydration
   B. Increased plasma volumes
   C. Overhydration
   D. Sunstroke

6. Congestive heart failure is the most common cause of:
   A. Overhydration
   B. Edema
   C. Dehydration
   D. Decreased capillary hydrostatic pressure

7. The kidney acts as the chief regulator of:
   A. Aldosterone
   B. Ingested liquids
   C. Perspiration
   D. Sodium in body fluids

8. Excess aldosterone leads to:
   A. Hypervolemia
   B. Hypovolemia
   C. Hypertension
   D. Hypotension

9. Which of the following is the most abundant body fluid in a young adult male?
   A. Intracellular fluid
   B. Interstitial fluid
   C. Plasma
   D. Blood

10. The average fluid intake per day is:
    A. 500 ml
    B. 750 ml
    C. 1000 ml
    D. 1500 ml

Matching

Select the most correct answer from column B for each statement in column A. (Only one answer is correct.)

Column A	Column B
_____ 11. Extracellular	A. Glucose
_____ 12. Intracellular	B. Inside cells
_____ 13. Nonelectrolyte	C. Homeostasis
_____ 14. Electrolyte	D. Stimulates production of urine
_____ 15. Diuretic	E. Plasma
_____ 16. Fluid balance	F. Fluid imbalance
_____ 17. Edema	G. Dehydration
_____ 18. Prolonged diarrhea	H. Overhydration
_____ 19. Rapid IV fluids	I. "Water-pushing" force
_____ 20. Capillary blood pressure	J. Table salt

CHAPTER 19

Acid-Base Balance

It has been established in previous chapters that an equilibrium between intracellular and extracellular fluid volume must exist for homeostasis to be maintained. Equally important to homeostasis is the chemical acid-base balance of the body fluids. The degree of acidity or alkalinity of a body fluid is expressed in pH value. The neutral point, where a fluid would be neither acid nor alkaline, is pH 7. Increasing acidity is expressed as less than 7, and increasing alkalinity is expressed as greater than 7. Examples of body fluids that are acidic are gastric juice (1.6) and urine (6.0). Blood, on the other hand, is considered alkaline with a pH of 7.45.

Buffers are substances that prevent a sharp change in the pH of a fluid when an acid or base is added to it. They are one of several mechanisms that are constantly monitoring the pH of fluids in the body. If, for any reason, these mechanisms do not function properly, a pH imbalance occurs. These two kinds of imbalances are known as alkalosis and acidosis.

Maintaining the acid-base balance of body fluids is a matter of vital importance. If this balance varies even slightly, necessary chemical and cellular reactions cannot occur. Your review of this chapter is necessary to understand the delicate fluid balance necessary to survival.

TOPICS FOR REVIEW

Before progressing to Chapter 20 you should have an understanding of the pH of body fluids and the mechanisms that control the pH of these fluids in the body. Your study should conclude with a review of the metabolic and respiratory types of pH imbalances.

pH OF BODY

Choose the correct term from the options given and write the letter in the answer blank.

(A) Acid (B) Base

_____ 1. Lower concentration of hydrogen ions than hydroxide ions

_____ 2. Higher concentration of hydrogen ions than hydroxide ions

_____ 3. Gastric juice

_____ 4. Saliva

_____ 5. Arterial blood

_____ 6. Venous blood

_____ 7. Baking soda

_____ 8. Beer

_____ 9. Ammonia

_____ 10. Pancreatic fluid

If you have had difficulty with this section, review pages 474-477.

MECHANISMS THAT CONTROL pH OF BODY FLUIDS pH IMBALANCES

Multiple Choice

Circle the correct choice.

11. When carbon dioxide enters the blood, it reacts with the enzyme carbonic anhydrase to form:
    A. Sodium bicarbonate
    B. Water and carbon dioxide
    C. Ammonium chloride
    D. Bicarbonate ion
    E. Carbonic acid

12. The lungs remove _______________ liters of carbonic acid each day.
    A. 10
    B. 15
    C. 20
    D. 25
    E. 30

13. When a buffer reacts with a strong acid it changes the strong acid to a:
    A. Weak acid
    B. Strong base
    C. Weak base
    D. Water
    E. None of the above

14. Which one of the following is *not* a change in the blood that results from the buffering of fixed acids in tissue capillaries?
   A. The amount of carbonic acid increases slightly.
   B. The amount of bicarbonate in blood decreases.
   C. The hydrogen ion concentration of blood increases slightly.
   D. The blood pH decreases slightly.
   E. All of the above are changes that result from the buffering of fixed acids in tissue capillaries.

15. The most abundant acid in the body is:
   A. HCl
   B. Lactic acid
   C. Carbonic acid
   D. Acetic acid
   E. Sulfuric acid

16. The normal ratio of sodium bicarbonate to carbonic acid in arterial blood is:
   A. 5:1
   B. 10:1
   C. 15:1
   D. 20:1
   E. None of the above

17. Which of the following would *not* be a consequence of holding your breath?
   A. The amount of carbonic acid in the blood increases.
   B. The blood pH decreases.
   C. The body develops an alkalosis.
   D. No carbon dioxide leaves the body.

18. Which of the following is *not* true of the kidneys?
   A. They can eliminate larger amounts of acid than the lungs.
   B. More bases than acids are usually excreted by the kidneys.
   C. If the kidneys fail, homeostasis of acid-base balance fails.
   D. They are the most effective regulators of blood pH.

19. The pH of the urine may be as low as:
   A. 1.6
   B. 2.5
   C. 3.2
   D. 4.8
   E. 7.4

20. In the distal tubule cells, the product of the reaction aided by carbonic anhydrase is:
   A. Water
   B. Carbon dioxide
   C. Water and carbon dioxide
   D. Hydrogen ions
   E. Carbonic acid

21. In the distal tubule, ________________ leaves the tubule cells and enters the blood capillaries.
   A. Carbon dioxide
   B. Water
   C. HCO_3
   D. NaH_2PO_4
   E. $NaHCO_3$

True or False

If the statement is true, write "T" in the answer blank. If the statement is false, correct the statement by circling the incorrect term and writing the correct term in the answer blank.

__________________ 22. The body has three mechanisms for regulating the pH of its fluids. They are the heart mechanism, the respiratory mechanism, and the urinary mechanism.

__________________ 23. Buffers consist of two kinds of substances and are, therefore, often called duobuffers.

__________________ 24. Ordinary baking soda is one of the main buffers of the normally occurring "fixed" acids in the blood.

__________________ 25. The accumulation of ketone bodies in the blood results from excessive metabolism of fats most often seen in uncontrolled type 1 diabetes.

__________________ 26. Anything that causes an excessive increase in respiration will in time produce acidosis.

__________________ 27. The lungs are the body's most effective regulator of blood pH.

__________________ 28. More acids than bases are usually excreted by the kidneys because more acids than bases usually enter the blood.

__________________ 29. Blood levels of sodium bicarbonate can be regulated by the lungs.

__________________ 30. Blood levels of carbonic acid can be regulated by the kidneys.

If you have had difficulty with this section, review pages 477-482.

pH IMBALANCES
METABOLIC AND RESPIRATORY DISTURBANCES
VOMITING

Write the letter of the correct term on the blank next to the appropriate definition.

A. Metabolic acidosis
B. Metabolic alkalosis
C. Respiratory acidosis
D. Respiratory alkalosis
E. Vomiting
F. Normal saline
G. Ketoacidosis
H. Hyperventilation
I. Hypersalivation
J. Anxiety

_____ 31. Emesis

_____ 32. Uncontrolled type 1 diabetes

_____ 33. Chloride-containing solution

_____ 34. Bicarbonate deficit

_____ 35. Present during emesis

_____ 36. Bicarbonate excess

_____ 37. Rapid breathing

_____ 38. Carbonic acid excess

_____ 39. Carbonic acid deficit

_____ 40. Hyperventilation syndrome

If you have had difficulty with this section, review pages 481-486.

UNSCRAMBLE THE WORDS

Take the circled letters, unscramble them, and fill in the statement.

41. **U L I F D S**

42. **E B T I A C N A O B R**

43. **A B S E**

44. **X F D E I**

45. **R O G H Y N E D**

How Sam the "stunt man" used his mattress.

46.

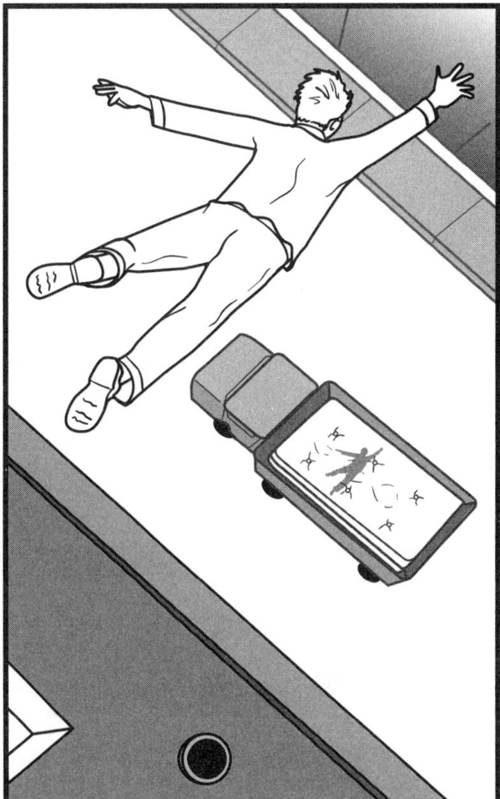

APPLYING WHAT YOU KNOW

47. Holly was pregnant and was experiencing repeated vomiting episodes for several days. Her doctor became concerned, admitted her to the hospital, and began intravenous administrations of normal saline. How will this help Holly?

48. Cara had a minor bladder infection. She had heard that this is often the result of the urine being less acidic than necessary, and that she should drink cranberry juice to correct the acid problem. She had no cranberry juice, so she decided to substitute orange juice. What was wrong with this substitution?

49. Mr. Almaguer has frequent bouts of hyperacidity of the stomach. Which will assist in neutralizing the acid more promptly; milk or Milk of Magnesia?

50. WORD FIND

Can you find 18 terms from this chapter in the box of letters? Words may be spelled top to bottom, bottom to top, right to left, left to right, or diagonally.

```
S I S A T S O E M O H P R G
E C N A L A B D I U L F E F
T S Y E N D I K W T I K A J
Y D M N D E J W L P T D J I
L D N O L H V W O U H D O I
O V E R H Y D R A T I O N S
R E I E E D E M A U R O R Q
T L M T C R U L R F S E O Y
C C U S Z A W E K A T N I X
E O Z O T T T A N A U N M F
L F K D P I O I W W Q L G Q
E N I L C O O H O W S B X S
N J X A L N F S U N L J J J
O C U V S A L G T I S C Z X
N I Z L L D Y X Q Q K D C D
```

ADH	Edema	Nonelectrolytes
Aldosterone	Electrolytes	Output
Anions	Fluid balance	Overhydration
Cations	Homeostasis	Sodium
Dehydration	Intake	Thirst
Diuretic	Kidneys	Water

DID YOU KNOW?

The brain is a 3-pound greedy organ that demands 17% of all cardiac output and 20% of all available oxygen.

English ships carried limes to protect the sailors from scurvy. American ships carried cranberries.

ACID/BASE BALANCE

Fill in the crossword puzzle.

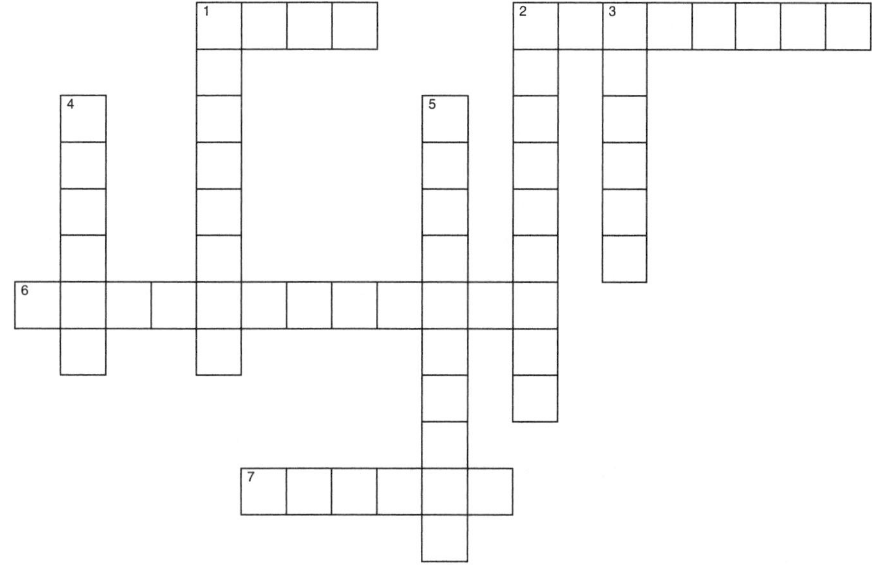

Across

1. Substance with a pH lower than 7.0
2. Acid-base imbalance
6. Results from the excessive metabolism of fats in uncontrolled diabetics (2 words)
7. Vomitus

Down

1. Substance with a pH higher than 7.0
2. Serious complication of vomiting
3. Emetic
4. Prevents a sharp change in the pH of fluids
5. Released as a waste product from working muscles (2 words)

CHECK YOUR KNOWLEDGE

Multiple Choice

Circle the correct answer.

1. A pH lower than 7.0 indicates:
   A. An acid solution
   B. An alkaline solution
   C. A lower concentration of hydrogen than hydroxide ions
   D. Both A and C

2. The overall pH range is expressed numerically on what is called a(n):
   A. pH calculator
   B. Acid-base numerator
   C. Logarithmic scale of 1–14
   D. Hydrogen-hydroxide value indicator

3. Chemical substances that prevent a sharp change in the pH of a fluid when an acid or base is added to it are called:
   A. Buffers
   B. Ketone bodies
   C. Enzymes
   D. Fixed acids

4. Lactic acid and other "fixed" acids are buffered by _________ in the blood.
   A. Hydrochloric acid
   B. Carbonic acid
   C. Carbon dioxide
   D. Sodium bicarbonate

5. Which of the following occurs during the vomit reflex?
   A. Hypersalivation
   B. Glottis opens
   C. Diaphragm relaxes
   D. Cardiac sphincter contracts

6. Which of the following is responsible for regulating pH of body fluids?
   A. Respiratory mechanism
   B. Urinary mechanism
   C. Buffer mechanism
   D. All of the above

7. Which of the following statements regarding metabolic disturbances is correct?
   A. Metabolic acidosis is a bicarbonate deficit.
   B. Metabolic alkalosis is a bicarbonate excess.
   C. Metabolic alkalosis is a complication of severe vomiting.
   D. All of the above are correct.

8. Which of the following statements regarding respiratory disturbances is correct?
   A. Depression of the respiratory center by drugs or disease can cause respiratory acidosis.
   B. Hyperventilation can result in respiratory alkalosis.
   C. Excess carbon dioxide in the arterial blood contributes to respiratory acidosis.
   D. All of the above are correct.

9. The key to acid-base balance is the:
   A. CO_2 ratio
   B. Buffer mechanism
   C. Ratio of respirations to blood pH levels
   D. Ratio of $NaHCO_3$ to H_2CO_3

10. A rare, but serious, complication of the medication Glucophage for type 2 diabetes is:
    A. Lactic acidosis
    B. Respiratory alkalosis
    C. Metabolic alkalosis
    D. None of the above

Matching

Select the most correct answer from column B for each statement in column A. (Only one answer is correct.)

Column A	Column B
_____ 11. Blood	A. Excessive fat metabolism
_____ 12. Gastric juice	B. Red blood cell enzyme
_____ 13. Aerobic respiration	C. Acid
_____ 14. "Fixed" acid	D. pH imbalance
_____ 15. Buffer	E. Lactic acid
_____ 16. Ketone bodies	F. Baking soda
_____ 17. Carbonic anhydrase	G. Alkaline
_____ 18. Acidosis	H. Respiratory acidosis
_____ 19. Hyperventilation	I. Cellular respiration
_____ 20. Emphysema	J. Respiratory alkalosis

CHAPTER 20

Reproductive Systems

The reproductive system consists of those organs that participate in perpetuating the species. It is a unique body system in that its organs differ between the two sexes and yet they work toward the same goal: creating a new life. Of interest also is the fact that this system is the only one not necessary to the survival of the individual, and yet survival of the species depends on its proper functioning. The male reproductive system is divided into the external genitals, the testes, the duct system, and accessory glands. The testes, or gonads, are considered essential organs because they produce the sex cells, sperm, that join with the female sex cells, ova, to form a new human being. They also secrete the male sex hormone, testosterone, which is responsible for the physical transformation of a boy to a man.

Sperm are formed in the testes by the seminiferous tubules. From there they enter a long narrow duct, the epididymis. They continue onward through the vas deferens into the ejaculatory duct, down the urethra, and out of the body. Throughout this journey, various glands secrete substances that add motility to the sperm and create a chemical environment conducive to reproduction.

The female reproductive system is truly extraordinary and diverse. It produces ova, receives the penis and sperm during intercourse, serves as the site of conception, houses and feeds the embryo during prenatal development, and nourishes the infant after birth.

Because of its diversity, the physiology of the female is generally considered to be more complex than that of the male. Much of the activity of this system revolves around the menstrual cycle and the monthly preparation that the female undergoes for a possible pregnancy.

The organs of the female system are divided into essential organs and accessory organs of reproduction. The essential organs of the female are the ovaries. Just as with the male, the essential organs of the female are referred to as the gonads. The gonads of both sexes produce the sex cells. In the male, the gonads produce the sperm and in the female they produce the ova. The gonads are also responsible for producing the hormones in each sex necessary for the appearance of the secondary sex characteristics.

The menstrual cycle of the female typically covers a period of 28 days. Each cycle consists of three phases: the menstrual period, the postmenstrual phase, and the premenstrual phase. Changes in the blood levels of the hormones that are responsible for the menstrual cycle also cause physical and emotional changes in the female. A knowledge of these phenomena and this system, in both the male and the female, are necessary to complete your understanding of the reproductive system.

TOPICS FOR REVIEW

Before progressing to Chapter 21 you should familiarize yourself with the structure and function of the organs of the male and female reproductive systems. Your review should include emphasis on the gross and microscopic structure of the testes and the production of sperm and testosterone. Your study should continue by tracing the pathway of a sperm cell from formation to expulsion from the body.

You should then familiarize yourself with the structure and function of the organs of the female reproductive system. Your review should include emphasis on the development of a mature ovum from ovarian follicles, and should additionally concentrate on the phases and occurrences in a typical 28-day menstrual cycle.

MALE REPRODUCTIVE SYSTEM STRUCTURAL PLAN

Match the term on the left with the proper selection on the right.

Group A

_____	1. Testes	A. Fertilized ovum
_____	2. Spermatozoa	B. Accessory organ
_____	3. Ova	C. Male sex cell
_____	4. Penis	D. Gonads
_____	5. Zygote	E. Gamete

Group B

_____	6. Testes	A. Cowper's gland
_____	7. Bulbourethral	B. Scrotum
_____	8. Asexual	C. Essential organ
_____	9. External genitalia	D. Single parent
_____	10. Prostate	E. Accessory organ

If you have had difficulty with this section, review pages 490-493.

TESTES

Multiple Choice

Circle the correct answer.

11. The testes are surrounded by a tough membrane called the:
    A. Ductus deferens
    B. Tunica albuginea
    C. Septum
    D. Seminiferous membrane

12. The ______________ lie near the septa that separate the lobules.
    A. Ductus deferens
    B. Sperm
    C. Interstitial cells
    D. Nerves

13. Sperm are found in the walls of the:
    A. Seminiferous tubule
    B. Interstitial cells
    C. Septum
    D. Blood vessels

14. An undescended testicle is called a(n):
    A. Orchidalgia
    B. Orchidorrhaphy
    C. Orchichorea
    D. Cryptorchidism

15. The structure(s) that produce(s) testosterone is (are) the:
    A. Seminiferous tubules
    B. Prostate gland
    C. Bulbourethral gland
    D. Pituitary gland
    E. Interstitial cells

16. The part of the sperm that contains genetic information that will be inherited is the:
    A. Tail
    B. Neck
    C. Middle piece
    D. Head
    E. Acrosome

17. Which one of the following is *not* a function of testosterone?
    A. It causes a deepening of the voice.
    B. It promotes the development of the male accessory glands.
    C. It has a stimulatory effect on protein catabolism.
    D. It causes greater muscular development and strength.

18. Sperm production is called:
    A. Spermatogonia
    B. Spermatids
    C. Spermatogenesis
    D. Spermatocyte

19. The section of the sperm that contains enzymes that enable it to break down the covering of the ovum and permit entry should contact occur is the:
    A. Acrosome
    B. Midpiece
    C. Tail
    D. Stem

20. Descent of the testes usually occurs about:
    A. Two months after birth
    B. Two months before birth
    C. Two months after conception
    D. Two years after birth
    E. None of the above

Completion

Fill in the blanks.

The (21) ____________________ are the gonads of the male. From puberty on, the seminiferous tubules are continuously forming (22) ____________________. Any of these cells may join with the female sex cell, the (23) ____________________, to become a new human being.

Another function of the testes is to secrete the male hormone (24) ____________________ which transforms a boy to a man. This hormone is secreted by the (25) __________________ __________________ of the testes. A good way to remember testosterone's functions is to think of it as "the (26) ______________________ hormone" and "the (27) ______________________ hormone."

If you have had difficulty with this section, review pages 493-498.

REPRODUCTIVE DUCTS
ACCESSORY OR SUPPORTIVE SEX GLANDS
EXTERNAL GENITALIA

Choose the correct term and write the letter in the space next to the appropriate definition below.

A. Epididymis
B. Vas deferens
C. Ejaculatory duct
D. Prepuce
E. Seminal vesicles
F. Prostate gland
G. Cowper's gland
H. Prostatectomy
I. Semen
J. Scrotum

_____ 28. Continuation of ducts that start in epididymis

_____ 29. Procedure performed for benign prostatic hypertrophy

_____ 30. Also known as "bulbourethral"

_____ 31. Narrow tube that lies along the top and behind the testes

_____ 32. Doughnut-shaped gland beneath bladder

_____ 33. Continuation of ductus deferens

_____ 34. Mixture of sperm and secretions of accessory sex glands

_____ 35. Contributes 60% of the seminal fluid volume

_____ 36. Removed during circumcision

_____ 37. External genitalia

If you have had difficulty with this section, review pages 497-499.

FEMALE REPRODUCTIVE SYSTEM STRUCTURAL PLAN

Match the term on the left with the proper selection on the right.

_____	38. Ovaries	A. External genitals
_____	39. Vagina	B. Accessory sex gland
_____	40. Bartholin	C. Accessory duct
_____	41. Vulva	D. Gonads
_____	42. Ova	E. Sex cells

Select the correct term from the options given and write the letter in the answer blank.

(A) External structure (B) Internal structure

_____ 43. Mons pubis

_____ 44. Vagina

_____ 45. Labia majora

_____ 46. Uterine tubes

_____ 47. Vestibule

_____ 48. Clitoris

_____ 49. Labia minora

_____ 50. Ovaries

If you have had difficulty with this section, review pages 499-501, 504 (Figure 20-9), and 507 (Figure 20-11).

OVARIES

Fill in the blanks.

The ovaries are the (51) ____________________ of the female. They have two main functions. The first is the production of the female sex cell. This process is called (52) ____________________. The specialized type of cell division that occurs during sexual cell reproduction is known as (53) ____________________. The ovum is the body's largest cell and has (54) ______________ ______________ the number of chromosomes found in other body cells. At the time of (55) ____________________, the sex cells from both parents fuse and (56) ____________________ chromosomes are united.

The second major function of the ovaries is to secrete the sex hormones (57) ____________________ and (58) ____________________. Estrogen is the sex hormone that causes the development and maintenance of the female (59) ______________ ______________ ______________. Progesterone acts with estrogen to help initiate the (60) ______________ ______________ in girls entering (61) ______________.

If you have had difficulty with this section, review pages 501-503.

FEMALE REPRODUCTIVE DUCTS

Select the correct term from the options given and write the letter in the answer blank.

(A) Uterine tubes (B) Uterus (C) Vagina

_____ 62. Ectopic pregnancy

_____ 63. Lining known as endometrium

_____ 64. Terminal end of birth canal

_____ 65. Site of menstruation

_____ 66. Approximately 4 inches in length

_____ 67. Consists of body, fundus, and cervix

_____ 68. Site of fertilization

_____ 69. Also known as "oviduct"

_____ 70. Entranceway for sperm

_____ 71. Total hysterectomy

If you have had difficulty with this section, review pages 503-505 and 510.

ACCESSORY OR SUPPORTIVE SEX GLANDS EXTERNAL GENITALS OF THE FEMALE

Match the term on the left with the proper selection on the right.

Group A

_____ 72. Bartholin's gland

_____ 73. Breasts

_____ 74. Alveoli

_____ 75. Lactiferous ducts

_____ 76. Areola

A. Colored area around nipple

B. Grapelike clusters of milk-secreting cells

C. Drain alveoli

D. Secretes lubricating fluid

E. Primarily fat tissue

Group B

_____ 77. Mons pubis

_____ 78. Labia majora

_____ 79. Clitoris

_____ 80. Vestibule

_____ 81. Episiotomy

A. "Large lips"

B. Area between labia minora

C. Surgical procedure

D. Composed of erectile tissue

E. Pad of fat over the symphysis pubis

If you have had difficulty with this section, review pages 505-506.

MENSTRUAL CYCLE

True or False

If the statement is true, insert "T" in the answer blank. If the statement is false, correct the statement by circling the incorrect term and writing the correct term in the answer blank.

____________________ 82. "Climacteric" is the scientific name for the beginning of the menses.

____________________ 83. As a general rule, several ovum mature each month during the 30–40 years that a woman has menstrual periods.

____________________ 84. Ovulation occurs 28 days before the next menstrual period begins.

____________________ 85. The first day of ovulation is considered the first day of the cycle.

____________________ 86. A woman's fertile period lasts only a few days out of each month.

____________________ 87. The control of the menstrual cycle lies in the posterior pituitary gland.

Matching

Write the letter of the correct hormone in the blank next to the appropriate description.

(A) FSH (B) LH

_____ 88. Ovulating hormone

_____ 89. Secreted during first days of menstrual cycle

_____ 90. Secreted after estrogen level of blood increases

_____ 91. Causes final maturation of follicle and ovum

_____ 92. Birth control pills suppress this hormone

If you have had difficulty with this section, review pages 506-512.

UNSCRAMBLE THE WORDS

93. **ULAVV**

94. **TSTSEE**

95. **MNSSEE**

96. **AIEIFMBR**

97. **CUERPPE**

Take the circled letters, unscramble them, and fill in the statement.

Where Kathleen displayed the flowers from her husband.

98.

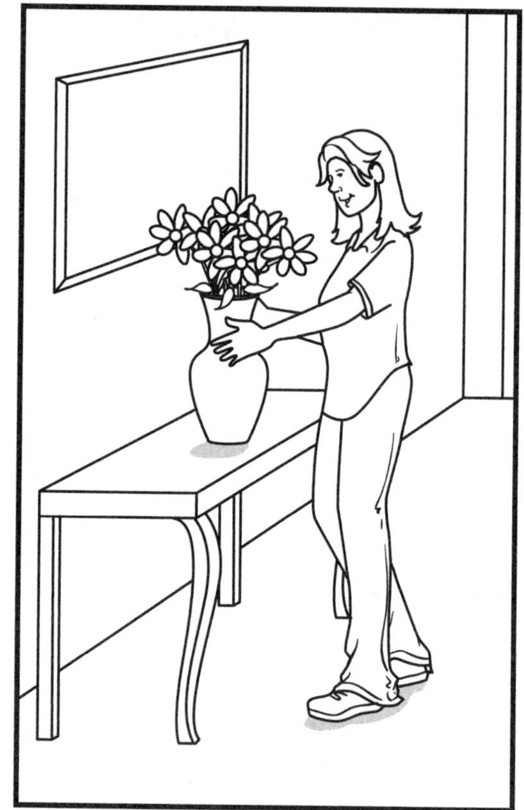

APPLYING WHAT YOU KNOW

99. Mr. Belinki is going into the hospital for the surgical removal of his testes. As a result of this surgery, will Mr. Belinki be impotent?

100. When baby Ross was born, the pediatrician discovered that his left testicle had not descended into the scrotum. If this situation is not corrected soon, might baby Ross be sterile or impotent?

101. Ms. Satin contracted gonorrhea. By the time she made an appointment to see her doctor, it had spread to her abdominal organs. How is this possible when gonorrhea is a disease of the reproductive system?

102. Mrs. Harlan was having a bilateral oophorectomy. Is this a sterilization procedure? Will she experience menopause?

103. Delceta had a total hysterectomy. Will she experience menopause?

104. WORD FIND

Can you find 18 terms from this chapter in the box of letters? Words may be spelled top to bottom, bottom to top, right to left, left to right, or diagonally.

```
M K O V I D U C T S E D H G
S E I R A V O I F U T G L L
I N H Z H M P M K O H I C W
D D V A S D E F E R E N S H
I O A C C I P J V E H Y D S
H M G R R B M N X F G Y I O
C E I O O E Z Y T I C S T E
R T N S T P S D D N O V A D
O R A O U W E B A I J S M Z
T I C M M E Y N E M D L R V
P U A E U D G M I E H I E H
Y M O T C E T A T S O R P B
R P E E R M N E G O R T S E
C O W P E R S I N X K E A P
```

Acrosome	Meiosis	Scrotum
Cowpers	Ovaries	Seminiferous
Cryptorchidism	Oviducts	Sperm
Endometrium	Penis	Spermatids
Epididymis	Pregnancy	Vagina
Estrogen	Prostatectomy	Vas deferens

DID YOU KNOW?

The testes produce approximately 50 million sperm per day. Every 2–3 months they produce enough cells to populate the entire earth.

There are an estimated 925,000 daily occurrences of STD transmission and 550,000 daily pregnancies worldwide.

REPRODUCTIVE SYSTEM

Fill in the crossword puzzle.

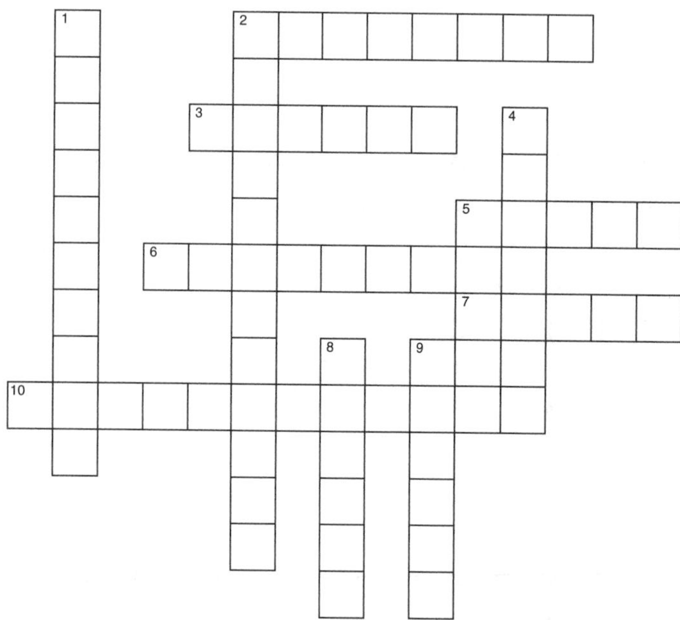

Across
2. Female erectile tissue
3. Colored area around nipple
5. Male reproductive fluid
6. Sex cells
7. External genitalia
10. Male sex hormone

Down
1. Failure to have a menstrual period
2. Surgical removal of foreskin
4. Foreskin
8. Menstrual period
9. Essential organs of reproduction

CHECK YOUR KNOWLEDGE

Multiple Choice

Circle the correct answer.

1. Which of the following is *not* an accessory organ of the male reproductive system?
   A. Gonads
   B. Prostate gland
   C. Scrotum
   D. Seminal vesicle

2. The acrosome:
   A. Contains the ATP to provide energy for the sperm
   B. Lies within the nucleus of the sperm
   C. Is responsible for sperm reproduction
   D. Contains enzymes that enable the sperm to enter the ovum

3. Which of the following contribute to the production of seminal fluid?
   A. Seminal vesicles
   B. Prostate gland
   C. Bulbourethral glands
   D. All of the above

4. Sperm mature and develop their ability to move or swim in the:
   A. Ductus deferens
   B. Ejaculatory duct
   C. Epididymis
   D. Cowper's glands

5. The bulbourethral glands:
   A. Are shaped like a doughnut
   B. Contribute 60% of the seminal fluid
   C. Secrete "pre-ejaculate"
   D. Pass through the inguinal canal as part of the spermatic cord

6. A mature ovum in its sac is sometimes called a(n):
   A. Graafian follicle
   B. Corpus luteum
   C. Oocyte
   D. Oogenesis

7. Progesterone:
   A. Initiates the first menstrual cycle
   B. Is produced by the corpus luteum
   C. Is responsible for the appearance of pubic hair and breast development
   D. All of the above

8. The external genitalia include all of the following *except:*
   A. Hymen
   B. Clitoris
   C. Lactiferous ducts
   D. Labia minora

9. Testosterone is produced by the:
   A. Interstitial cells
   B. Seminiferous tubules
   C. Process of meiosis
   D. Tunica albuginea

10. Which of the following analogous features of the reproductive systems is correct?
    A. Ovaries to testes
    B. Estrogen and progesterone to testosterone
    C. Clitoris and vulva to penis and scrotum
    D. All of the above

Matching

Select the most correct answer from column B for each statement in column A. (Only one answer is correct.)

Column A	Column B
_____ 11. Sex cells	A. Spermatogonia
_____ 12. Sperm stem cells	B. FSH
_____ 13. Testosterone	C. Gametes
_____ 14. Penis	D. Menarche
_____ 15. Scrotum	E. LH
_____ 16. Ovulating hormone	F. Male external genitalia
_____ 17. Sperm formation	G. Prepuce
_____ 18. Menses	H. Masculinizes
_____ 19. Breasts	I. Female external genitalia
_____ 20. Vestibule	J. Areola

MALE REPRODUCTIVE ORGANS

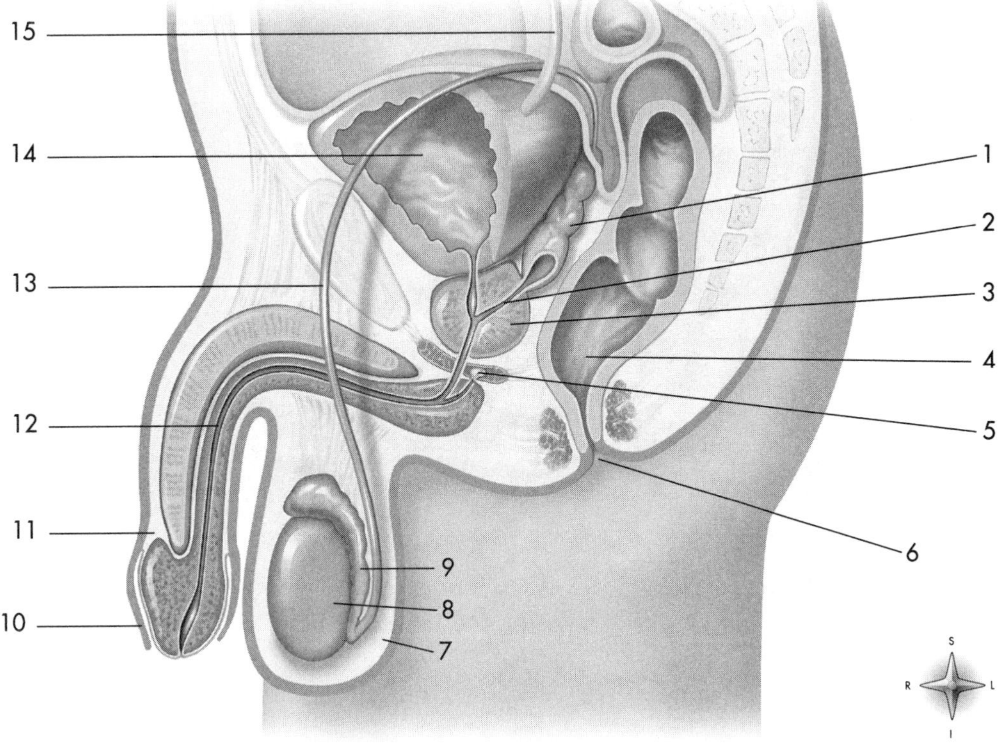

1. ______________________
2. ______________________
3. ______________________
4. ______________________
5. ______________________
6. ______________________
7. ______________________
8. ______________________
9. ______________________
10. ______________________
11. ______________________
12. ______________________
13. ______________________
14. ______________________
15. ______________________

TUBULES OF TESTIS AND EPIDIDYMIS

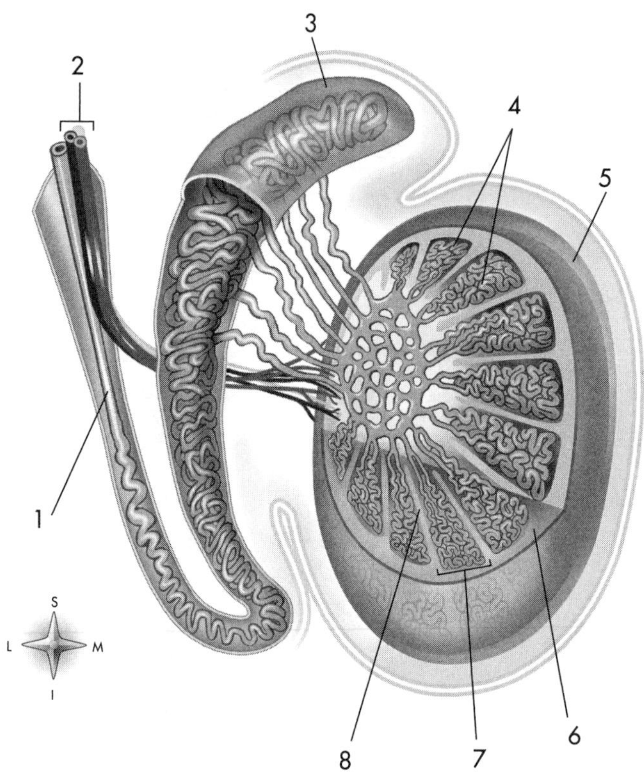

1. ______________________
2. ______________________
3. ______________________
4. ______________________
5. ______________________
6. ______________________
7. ______________________
8. ______________________

VULVA

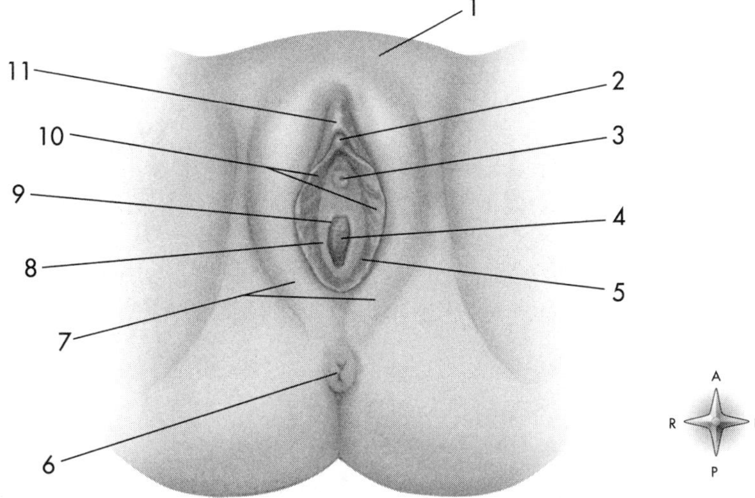

1. ______________________
2. ______________________
3. ______________________
4. ______________________
5. ______________________
6. ______________________
7. ______________________
8. ______________________
9. ______________________
10. ______________________
11. ______________________

BREAST

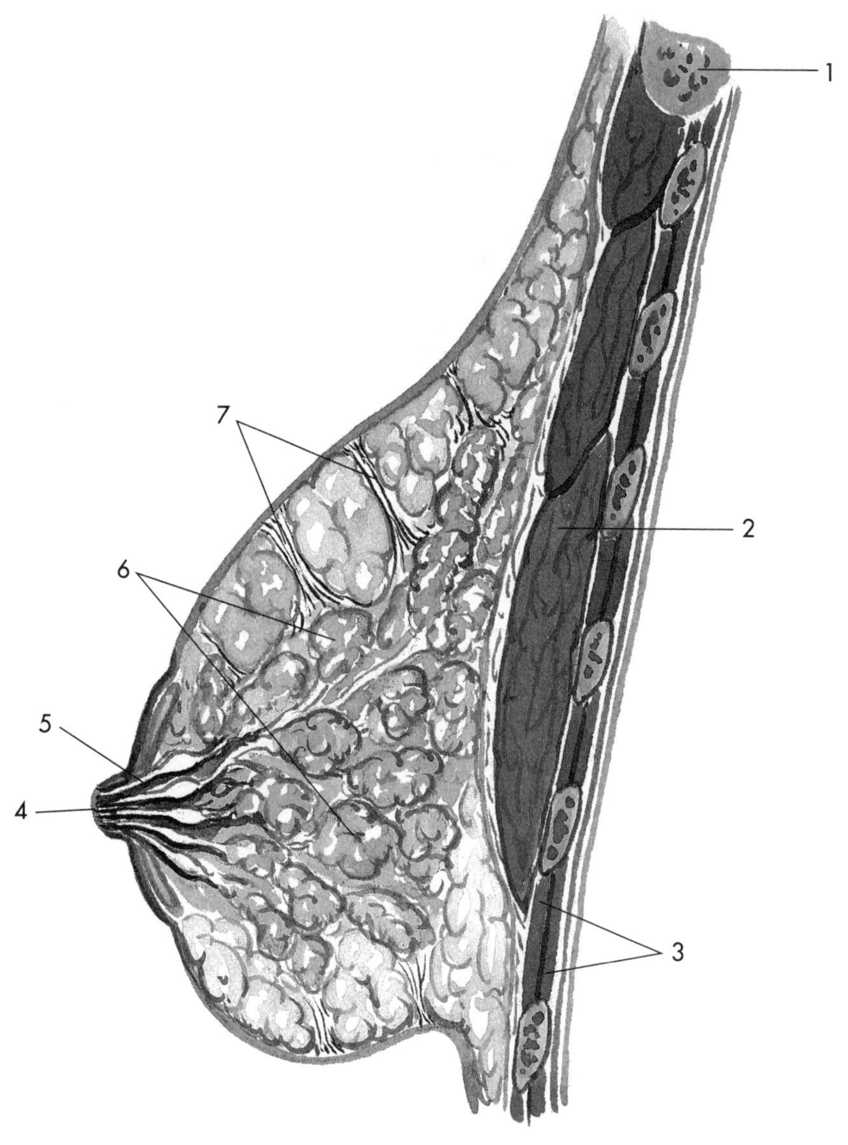

1. ______________________
2. ______________________
3. ______________________
4. ______________________
5. ______________________
6. ______________________
7. ______________________

FEMALE PELVIS

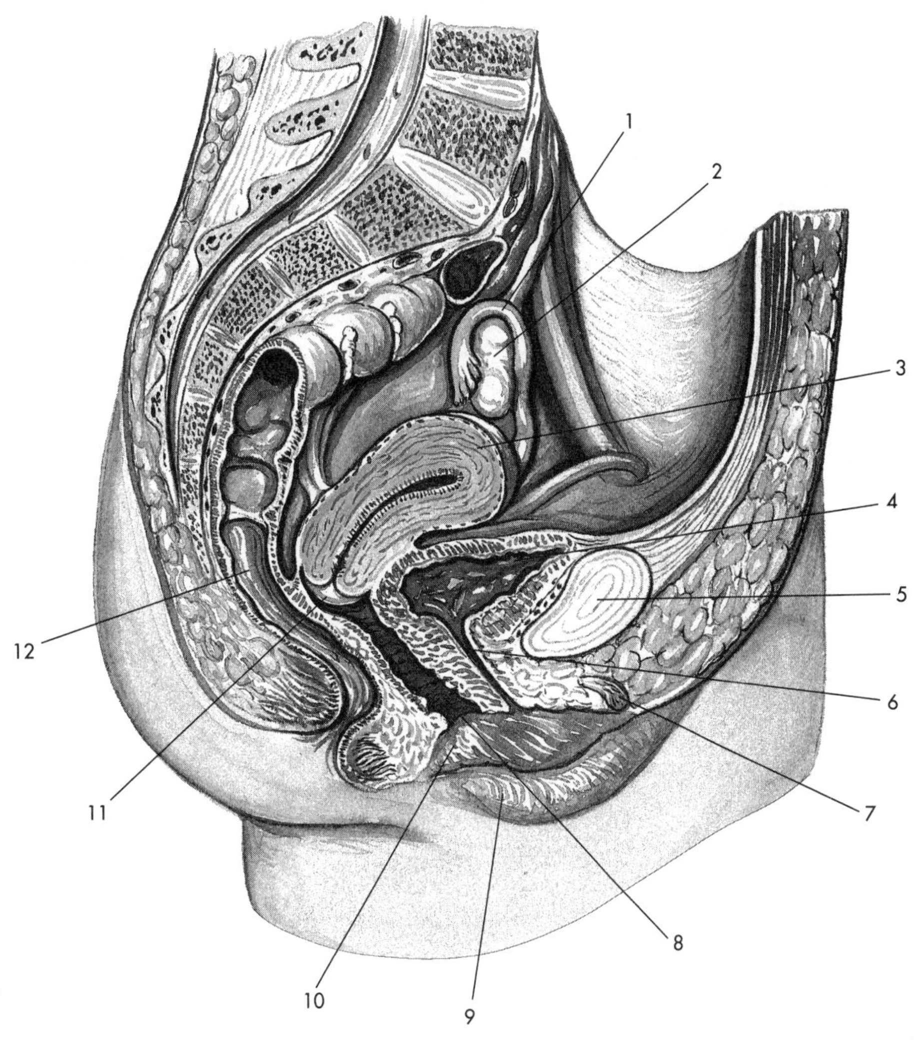

1. ______________________
2. ______________________
3. ______________________
4. ______________________
5. ______________________
6. ______________________
7. ______________________
8. ______________________
9. ______________________
10. ______________________
11. ______________________
12. ______________________

UTERUS AND ADJACENT STRUCTURES

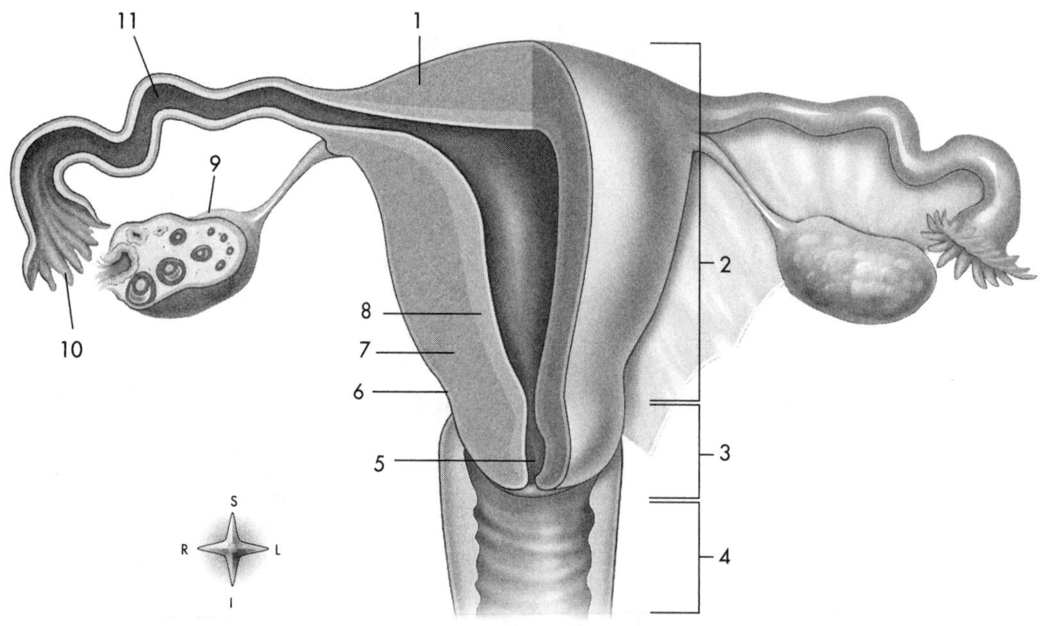

1. ______________________
2. ______________________
3. ______________________
4. ______________________
5. ______________________
6. ______________________
7. ______________________
8. ______________________
9. ______________________
10. ______________________
11. ______________________

CHAPTER 21

Growth and Development

Millions of fragile microscopic sperm swim against numerous obstacles to reach the ova and create a new life. At birth, the newborn will fill his lungs with air and cry lustily, signaling to the world that he is ready to begin the cycle of life. This cycle will be marked by ongoing changes, periodic physical growth, and continuous development.

This chapter reviews the more significant events that occur in the normal growth and development of an individual from conception to death. Realizing that each individual is unique, we nonetheless can discover, amid all the complexities of humanity, some constants that are understandable and predictable.

A knowledge of human growth and development is essential in understanding the commonalties that influence individuals as they pass through the cycle of life.

TOPICS FOR REVIEW

Your review of this chapter should include an understanding of the concept of development as a biological process. You should familiarize yourself with the major developmental changes from conception through older adulthood. Your study should conclude with a review of the effects of aging on the body systems.

PRENATAL PERIOD

Completion

Fill in the blanks.

The prenatal stage of development begins at the time of (1) ________________ and continues until (2) ________________. The science of the development of an individual before birth is called (3) ________________.

Fertilization takes place in the outer third of the (4) ________________. The fertilized ovum or (5) ________________ begins to divide and in approximately 3 days forms a solid mass called a (6) ________________. By the time it enters the uterus, it is a hollow ball of cells called a (7) ________________.

As it continues to develop, it forms a structure with two cavities. The (8) ____________ ____________ will become a fluid-filled sac for the embryo. The (9) ________________ will develop into an important fetal membrane in the (10) ________________.

Matching

Choose the correct term and write the letter in the space next to the appropriate definition below.

A. Laparoscope
B. Gestation
C. Antenatal
D. Histogenesis
E. Quickening
F. Endoderm
G. In vitro
H. Parturition
I. Embryonic phase
J. Ultrasonogram

_____ 11. "Within a glass"

_____ 12. Inside germ layer

_____ 13. Before birth

_____ 14. Length of pregnancy

_____ 15. Fiberoptic viewing instrument

_____ 16. Process of birth

_____ 17. First fetal movement

_____ 18. Study of how the primary germ layers develop into many different kinds of tissues

_____ 19. Fertilization until the end of the eighth week of gestation

_____ 20. Monitors the progress of the developing fetus.

If you have had difficulty with this section, review pages 520-530 and 532.

POSTNATAL PERIOD

Multiple Choice

Circle the correct answer.

21. During the postnatal period:
    A. The head becomes proportionately smaller
    B. Thoracic and abdominal contours change from round to elliptical
    C. The legs become proportionately longer
    D. The trunk becomes proportionately shorter
    E. All of the above

22. The period of infancy starts at birth and lasts about:
    A. 4 weeks
    B. 4 months
    C. 10 weeks
    D. 12 months
    E. 18 months

23. The lumbar curvature of the spine appears ____________ months after birth.
    A. 1–10
    B. 5–8
    C. 8–12
    D. 11–15
    E. 12–18

24. During the first 4 months the birth weight will:
    A. Double
    B. Triple
    C. Quadruple
    D. None of the above

25. At the end of the first year, the weight of the baby will have:
    A. Doubled
    B. Tripled
    C. Quadrupled
    D. None of the above

26. The infant is capable of following a moving object with its eyes at:
    A. 2 days
    B. 2 weeks
    C. 2 months
    D. 4 months
    E. 10 months

27. The infant can lift its head and raise its chest at:
    A. 2 months
    B. 3 months
    C. 4 months
    D. 10 months

28. The infant can crawl at the age of:
    A. 2 months
    B. 3 months
    C. 4 months
    D. 10 months
    E. 12 months

29. The infant can stand alone at the age of:
    A. 2 months
    B. 3 months
    C. 4 months
    D. 10 months
    E. 12 months

30. The permanent teeth, with the exception of the third molar, have all erupted by age _______ years.
    A. 6
    B. 8
    C. 12
    D. 14
    E. None of the above

31. Puberty starts at age ______________ years in boys.
    A. 10–13
    B. 12–14
    C. 14–16
    D. None of the above

32. Most girls begin breast development at about age:
    A. 8
    B. 9
    C. 10
    D. 11
    E. 12

33. The growth spurt is generally complete by age ___________ in males.
    A. 14
    B. 15
    C. 16
    D. 18

34. An average age at which girls begin to menstruate is __________ years.
    A. 10–12
    B. 11–12
    C. 12–13
    D. 13–14
    E. 14–15

35. The first sign of puberty in boys is:
    A. Facial hair
    B. Increased muscle mass
    C. Pubic hair
    D. Deepening of the voice
    E. Increased testicular enlargement

Matching

Write the letter of the correct word in the blank next to the appropriate definition.

A. Neonatology
B. Neonatal
C. Adolescence
D. Deciduous
E. Puberty
F. Postnatal
G. Infancy
H. Childhood
I. Senescence

_____ 36. Begins at birth and lasts until death

_____ 37. Concerned with the diagnosis and treatment of disorders of the newborn

_____ 38. Teenage years

_____ 39. From the end of infancy to puberty

_____ 40. Baby teeth

_____ 41. First 4 weeks of infancy

_____ 42. Secondary sexual characteristics occur

_____ 43. Begins at birth and lasts about 18 months

_____ 44. Older adulthood

If you have had difficulty with this section, review pages 530-536.

EFFECTS OF AGING

Fill in the blanks.

45. Old bones develop indistinct and shaggy margins with spurs, a process called ____________________.
46. A degenerative joint disease common in the aged is ____________________.
47. The number of __________________________ units in the kidney decreases by almost 50% between the ages of 30 and 75.
48. In older adulthood, respiratory efficiency decreases, and a condition known as ____________________ __________________ results.
49. Fatty deposits accumulate in blood vessels as we age, and the result is ____________________________, which narrows the passageway for the flow of blood.
50. Hardening of the arteries or ___________________________ occurs during the aging process.
51. Another term for high blood pressure is ___________________________.
52. Hardening of the lens is ___________________________.
53. If the lens becomes cloudy and impairs vision, it is called a ___________________________.
54. _____________________________ causes an increase in the pressure within the eyeball and may result in blindness.

If you have had difficulty with this section, review pages 536-540.

UNSCRAMBLE THE WORDS

Take the circled letters, unscramble them, and fill in the statement.

55. **ANNFCYI**

56. **NAALTTSOP**

57. **OGSSNEGRAONEI**

58. **GTEYZO**

59. **HDOOLHCID**

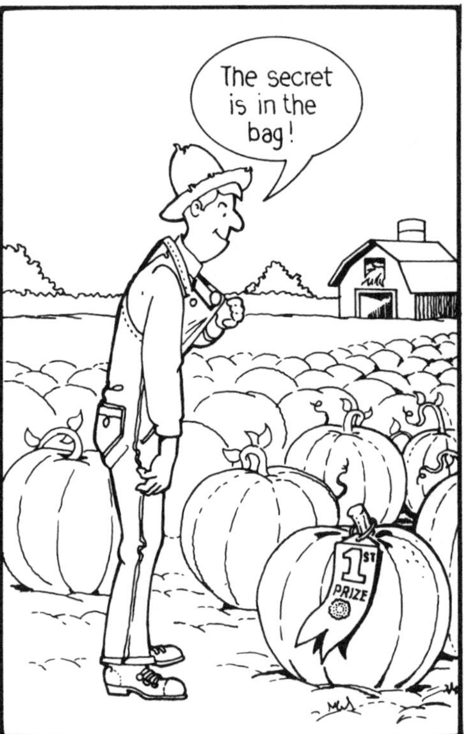

The secret to Farmer Brown's prize pumpkin crop.

60.

APPLYING WHAT YOU KNOW

61. Heather's mother told the pediatrician during her 1-year visit that Heather had tripled her birth weight, was crawling actively, and could stand alone. Is Heather's development normal, retarded, or advanced?

62. Becky is 70 years old. She has always enjoyed food and has had a hearty appetite. Lately, however, she has complained that food "just doesn't taste as good anymore." What might be a possible explanation?

63. Mr. Altman, age 68, has noticed hearing problems, but only under certain circumstances. He has difficulty with certain tones, especially high or low tones, but has no problem with everyday conversation. What might be a possible explanation?

64. WORD FIND

Can you find 14 terms from the chapter in the box of letters? Words may be spelled top to bottom, bottom to top, right to left, left to right, or diagonally.

```
F T P N O I T A T S E G K F U
Z E P O C S O R A P A L H E A
E O R I L T O H H O C J V J T
C M V T N T I M L N L Z P U O
M A B I I F R M R E D O T C E
H Q C R D L A M E S O D E R M
N N M U Y U I N M F O W G O P
K N V T C O C Z C H H F R C N
H G Y R Y K L T A Y D U C V P
L A T A N T S O P T L U N Q G
Q N K P Y Y S W G A I K E M T
U G P Q N H O Y X Y H O Z B N
I Y T R E B U P L A C E N T A
```

Childhood	Infancy	Parturition
Ectoderm	Laparoscope	Placenta
Embryology	Mesoderm	Postnatal
Fertilization	Morula	Puberty
Gestation	Oviduct	

DID YOU KNOW?

Brain cells do not regenerate. One beer permanently destroys 10,000 cells.

A 3-week old embryo is no larger than a sesame seed. A 1-month old fetus' body is no heavier than an envelope and a sheet of paper. Its hand is no bigger than a teardrop.

GROWTH/DEVELOPMENT

Fill in the crossword puzzle.

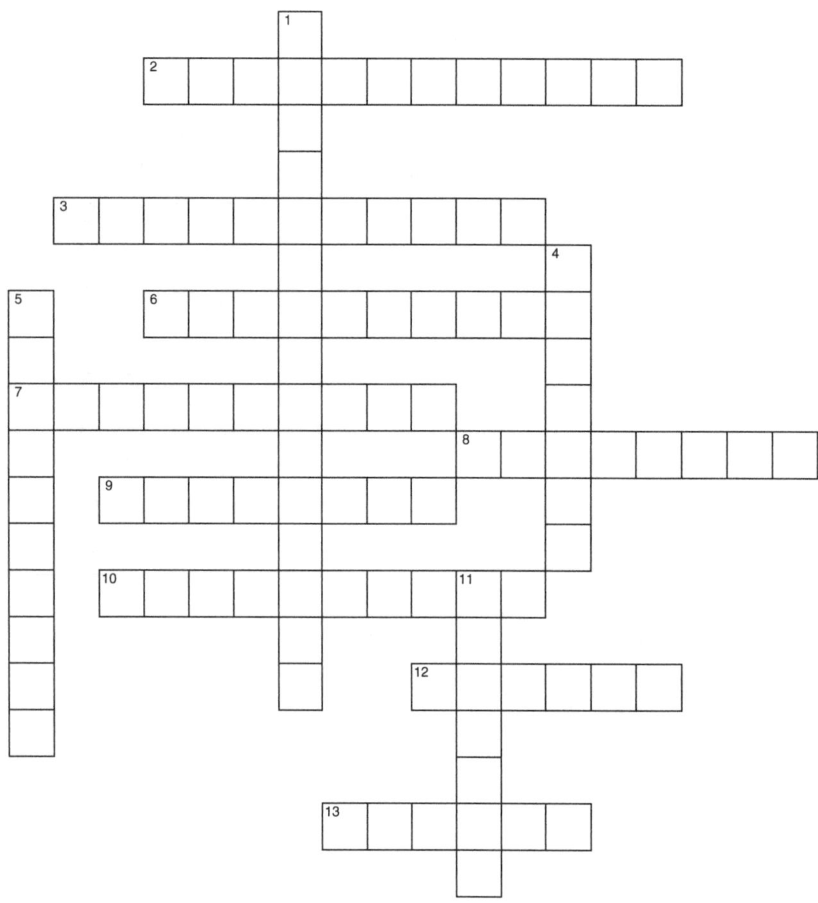

Across

2. Study of how germ layers develop into tissues
3. Process of birth
6. Name of zygote after implantation
7. Science of the development of the individual before birth
8. Eye disease marked by increased pressure in the eyeball
9. Cloudy lens
10. Old age
12. Name of zygote after 3 days
13. Fertilized ovum

Down

1. Fatty deposit buildup on walls of arteries
4. First 4 weeks of infancy
5. Hardening of the lens
11. Will develop into a fetal membrane in the placenta

CHECK YOUR KNOWLEDGE

Multiple Choice

Circle the correct answer.

1. The prenatal period begins:
   A. After implantation
   B. 4 weeks after gestation
   C. At conception
   D. 10 days after conception

2. By the time the developing embryo reaches the uterus, it is a:
   A. Morula
   B. Zygote
   C. Fetus
   D. Blastocyst

3. The chorion develops into the:
   A. Morula
   B. Zygote
   C. Fetus
   D. Placenta

4. Fertilization most often occurs in the:
   A. Outer one-third of the oviduct
   B. Inner one-third of the oviduct
   C. Uterus
   D. Vagina

5. The embryonic phase of development extends from fertilization until the end of week _______ of gestation.
   A. 2
   B. 4
   C. 6
   D. 8

6. The primary germ layers include the:
   A. Endoderm
   B. Ectoderm
   C. Mesoderm
   D. All of the above

7. The stage of labor that begins from the onset of uterine contractions until dilation of the cervix is complete is called:
   A. Parturition
   B. Transition
   C. Stage one
   D. Stage two

8. All organ systems are complete and in place by:
   A. 4 months of gestation
   B. 35 days of gestation
   C. 7 months of gestation
   D. 8 months of gestation

9. The initial stimulus to breathe when an infant is born results from the:
   A. Doctor shocking the baby by slapping the buttocks
   B. Cold new environment shocking the respiratory system
   C. Increasing amounts of carbon dioxide that accumulate in the blood after the umbilical cord is cut following delivery
   D. Baby's sudden change of position after delivery

10. Adulthood is characterized by:
    A. A period of rapid growth
    B. Maintenance of existing body tissues
    C. Senescence
    D. None of the above

Matching

Select the most correct answer from column B for each statement in column A. (Only one answer is correct.)

Column A	Column B
____ 11. Embryology	A. Study of aging
____ 12. Zygote	B. First 18 months of life
____ 13. Gestation period	C. Trimesters
____ 14. Older adult	D. Fetal movement
____ 15. Teratogens	E. Prenatal science
____ 16. Quickening	F. "Old eye"
____ 17. Lipping	G. Fertilized ovum
____ 18. Presbyopia	H. Factors that cause birth defects
____ 19. Gerontology	I. Senescence
____ 20. Infancy	J. Bone spurs

FERTILIZATION AND IMPLANTATION

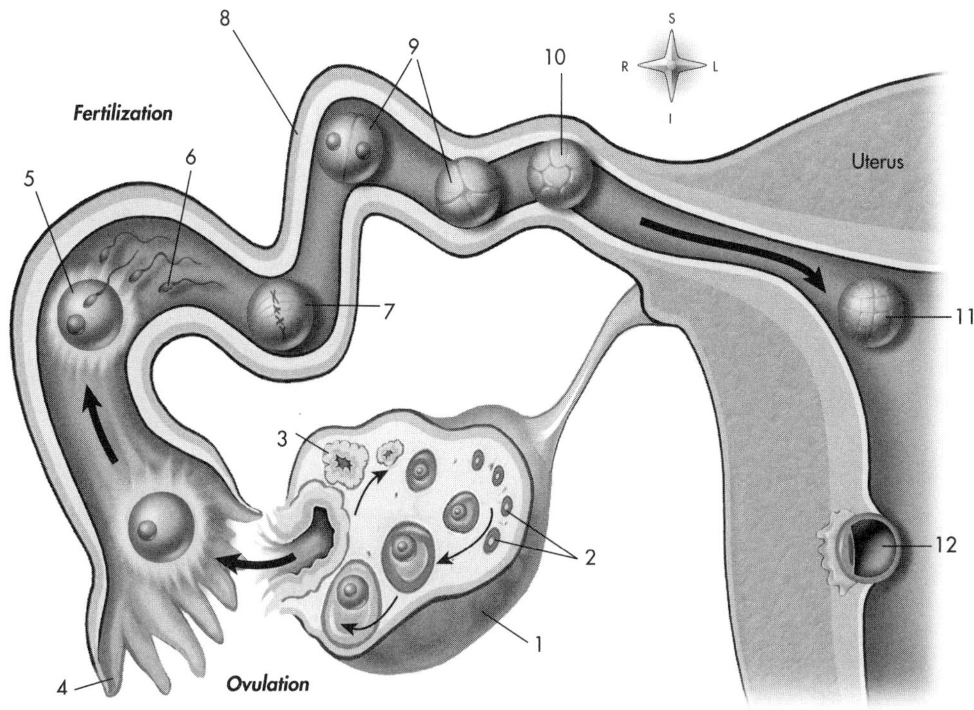

1. ______________________
2. ______________________
3. ______________________
4. ______________________
5. ______________________
6. ______________________
7. ______________________
8. ______________________
9. ______________________
10. ______________________
11. ______________________
12. ______________________

Answer Key

CHAPTER 1
AN INTRODUCTION TO THE STRUCTURE AND FUNCTION OF THE BODY

Matching
1. D, p. 4
2. E, p. 4
3. A, p. 4
4. C, p. 4
5. B, p. 6

Matching
6. C, p. 6
7. A, p. 6
8. E, p. 6
9. D, p. 6
10. B, p. 6

Crossword
11. Superior
12. Inferior
13. Transverse
14. Ventral
15. Lateral
16. Medial
17. Distal

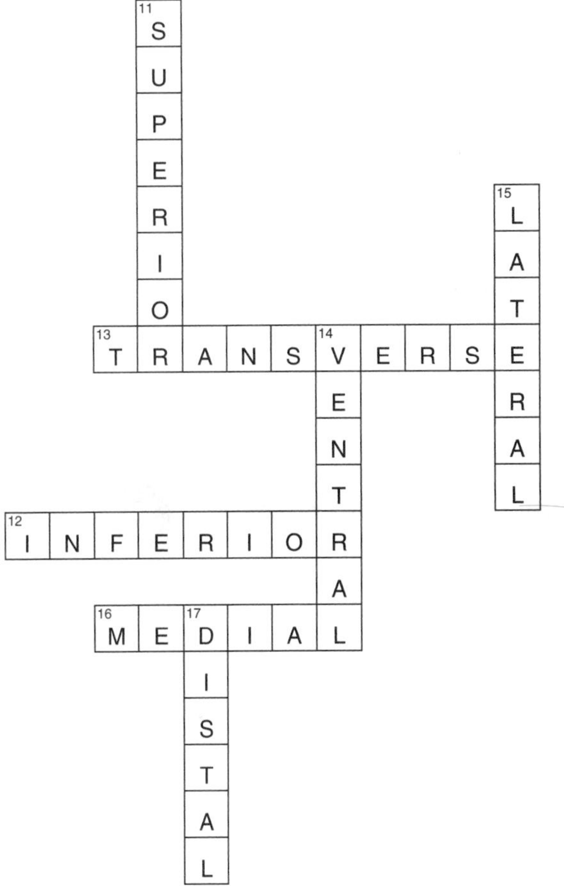

Did you notice that the answers were arranged as they appear on the human body?

Circle the correct answer

18. Inferior, p. 6
19. Anterior, p. 7
20. Lateral, p. 7
21. Proximal, p. 9
22. Superficial, p. 9
23. Equal, p. 9
24. Anterior and posterior, p. 9
25. Upper and lower, p. 9
26. Frontal, p. 9

Select the correct term

27. A, p. 10
28. B, p. 10
29. A, p. 10
30. A, p. 10
31. A, p. 10
32. B, p. 10
33. A, p. 10

Circle the one that does not belong

34. Extremities (all others are part of the axial portions)
35. Cephalic (all others are part of the arm)
36. Plantar (all others are part of the face)
37. Carpal (all others are part of the leg or foot)
38. Tarsal (all others are part of the skull)

Fill in the blanks

39. Survival, p. 13
40. Internal environment, p. 13
41. Feedback loop, p. 13
42. Negative, positive, p. 15
43. Stabilize, p. 15
44. Stimulatory, p. 15
45. Developmental processes, p. 17
46. Aging processes, p. 17

Applying what you know

47. #1 on diagram
48. #2 on diagram
49. #3 on diagram

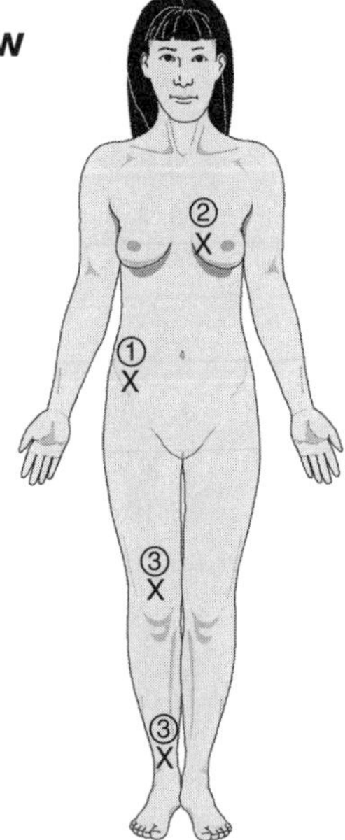

50. WORD FIND

N	H	L	T	E	B	W	N	G	N	M	M	Y	X	A
O	O	H	A	V	U	U	C	L	W	E	P	N	G	L
I	M	U	N	I	T	S	A	I	D	E	M	W	A	L
T	E	R	T	V	C	T	S	I	C	J	S	R	T	K
A	O	N	O	P	T	I	A	I	W	A	T	Y	R	H
Z	S	Q	S	I	R	L	F	A	T	N	R	G	O	W
I	T	W	G	P	R	O	I	R	E	T	S	O	P	F
N	A	A	Z	J	E	E	X	V	E	E	H	L	H	Z
A	S	N	L	M	C	T	P	I	C	P	D	O	Y	T
G	I	C	A	Y	U	O	X	U	M	N	U	I	V	P
R	S	M	R	T	N	U	K	B	S	A	Y	S	V	M
O	R	C	U	R	O	I	R	B	S	Q	L	Y	U	G
L	H	X	E	M	P	M	E	T	S	Y	S	H	V	S
U	W	L	L	Q	D	U	Y	Y	N	E	E	P	J	B
Q	N	Z	P	K	D	B	O	D	C	G	I	N	J	A

Check your knowledge

Multiple choice

1. A, p. 13
2. D, p. 11
3. B, p. 10
4. D, p. 9
5. A, p. 3
6. C, p. 10
7. C, p. 6
8. A, p. 9
9. C, p. 10
10. B, p. 11
11. D, p. 11
12. B, p. 10
13. C, p. 4
14. A, p. 9
15. D, p. 9
16. C, p. 6
17. D, p. 14
18. D, p. 9
19. A, p. 14
20. C, p. 7

Matching

21. F, p. 7
22. B, p. 15
23. J, p. 9
24. G, p. 3
25. H, p. 9
26. C, p. 10
27. D, p. 14
28. I, p. 7
29. A, p. 9
30. E, p. 5

Fill in the blanks

31. Scientific method
32. Hypothesis
33. Experimentation
34. Test group
35. Control group

Dorsal and ventral body cavities

1. Cranial cavity
2. Spinal cavity
3. Thoracic cavity
4. Mediastinum
5. Abdominal cavity
6. Pelvic cavity

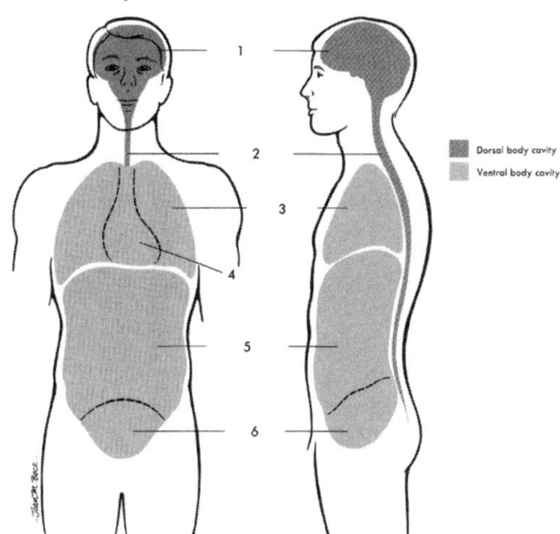

Directions and planes of the body

1. Superior
2. Proximal
3. Posterior (dorsal)
4. Anterior (ventral)
5. Inferior
6. Sagittal plane
7. Frontal plane
8. Lateral

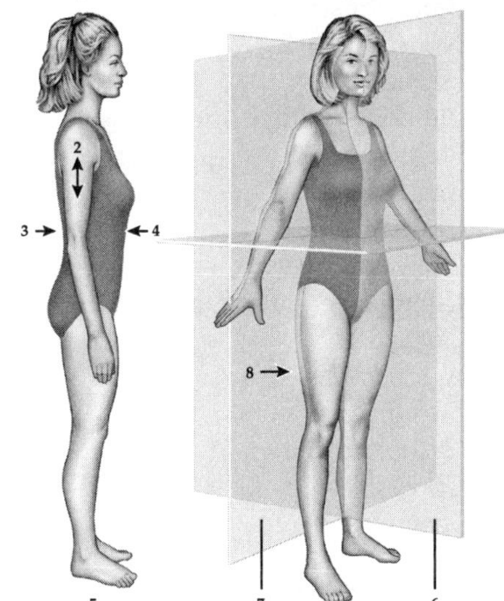

Regions of the abdomen

1. Epigastric region
2. Left hypochondriac region
3. Umbilical region
4. Left lumbar region
5. Left iliac (inguinal) region
6. Hypogastric region
7. Right iliac (inguinal) region
8. Right lumbar region
9. Right hypochondriac region

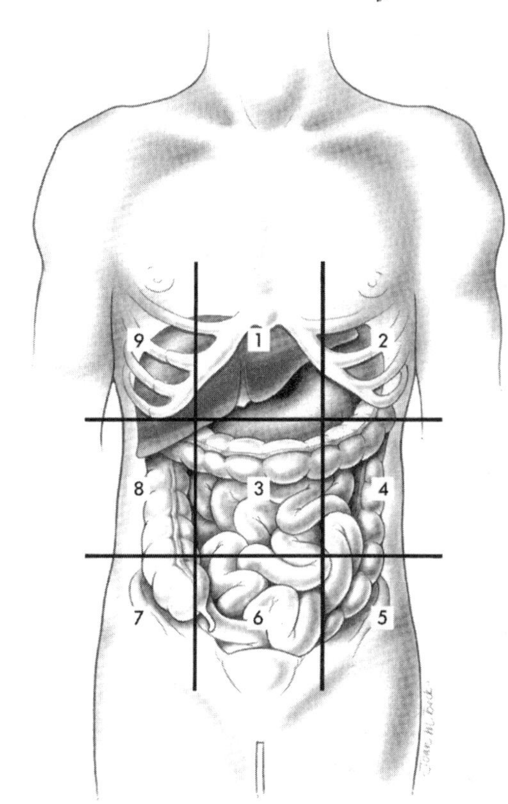

CHAPTER 2 CHEMISTRY OF LIFE

Multiple choice

1. C, p. 23
2. B, p. 24
3. C, p. 24
4. A, p. 24
5. D, p. 24
6. C, p. 25
7. A, p. 25

True or false

8. T, p. 23
9. molecules, p. 23
10. uncharged neutrons, p. 24
11. T, p. 24
12. T, p. 25

Multiple choice

13. C, p. 25
14. B, p. 25
15. A, p. 26
16. B, p. 26
17. A, p. 25
18. C, p. 25

Matching

19. H, p. 27
20. B, p. 27
21. E, p. 27
22. A, p. 27
23. G, p. 27
24. L, p. 27
25. J, p. 28
26. C, p. 28
27. D, p. 29
28. F, p. 29
29. K, p. 29
30. I, p. 29

Select the best answer

31. A, p. 31
32. B, p. 31
33. D, p. 35
34. B, p. 33
35. C, p. 33
36. A, p. 31
37. A, p. 31
38. B, p. 33
39. C, p. 33
40. D, p. 35

Crossword

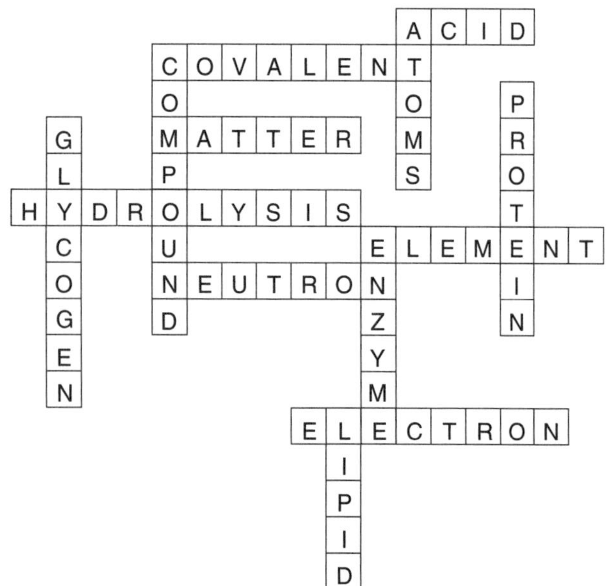

Unscramble the words

41. Matter
42. Elements
43. Molecules
44. Organic
45. Electrolyte
46. Energy

Applying what you know

47. Some fats can become solid at room temperature, such as the fat in butter and lard.
48. Radioactive isotopes will be used to measure Carol's thyroid activity. A diagnosis of hyperthyroidism or hypothyroidism will be based upon how rapidly or slowly the thyroid absorbs the radioactive iodine and emits radiation.

49. WORD FIND

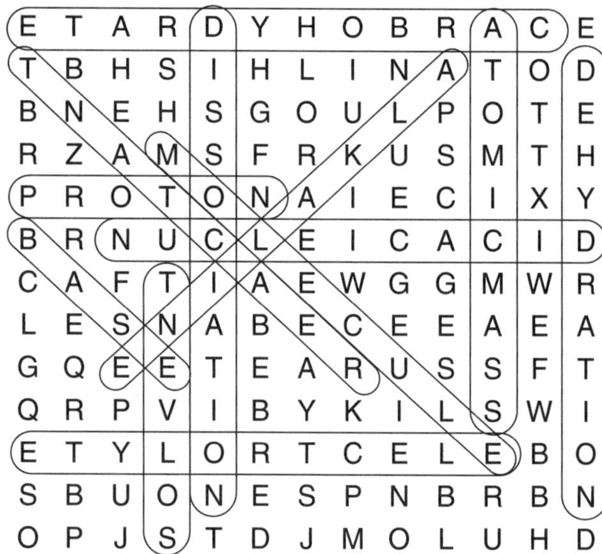

Check your knowledge

1. Biochemistry, p. 23
2. Neutrons, p. 23
3. Higher, p. 24
4. Elements; compounds, p. 24
5. Stable, p. 25
6. Ion, p. 25
7. Inorganic, p. 27
8. Dehydration synthesis, p. 27
9. Chemical equation, p. 28
10. CO_2, p. 29
11. Acids, p. 29
12. Buffers, p. 30
13. Carbohydrate, p. 31
14. Cholesterol, p. 33
15. Structural, p. 34

CHAPTER 3
CELLS AND TISSUES

Matching

Group A
1. C, p. 44
2. E, p. 44
3. A, p. 44
4. B, p. 44
5. D, p. 48

Group B
6. D, p. 45
7. E, p. 45
8. A, p. 47
9. B, p. 48
10. C, p. 46

Fill in the blanks
11. Organelles, p. 45
12. Tissue typing, p. 45
13. Cilia, p. 48
14. Aerobic; cellular respiration, p. 48
15. Ribosomes, p. 45
16. Mitochondria, p. 48
17. Lysosomes, p. 48
18. Golgi apparatus, p. 47
19. Centrioles, p. 48
20. Chromatin granules, p. 48

Circle the correct choice
21. A, p. 50
22. D, p. 50
23. B, p. 50
24. D, p. 51
25. C, p. 51
26. A, p. 51
27. B, p. 51
28. C, p. 52
29. D, p. 52
30. A, p. 53
31. B, p. 54
32. A, p. 54

Circle the one that does not belong
33. Uracil (RNA contains the base uracil, not DNA)
34. Telophase (the others are complementary base pairings of DNA)
35. Anaphase (the others refer to genes and heredity)
36. Thymine (the others refer to RNA)
37. Interphase (the others refer to translation)
38. Prophase (the others refer to anaphase)
39. Prophase (the others refer to interphase)
40. Metaphase (the others refer to telophase)
41. Gene (the others refer to stages of cell division)

42. Fill the missing areas

TISSUE	LOCATION	FUNCTION
Epithelial		
1.	1A.	1A. Absorption by diffusion of respiratory gases between alveolar air and blood
	1B.	1B. Absorption by diffusion, filtration, and osmosis
2.	2A. Surface of lining of mouth and esophagus	2A.
	2B. Surface of skin	2B.
3.	3. Surface layer of lining of stomach, intestines, and parts of respiratory tract	3.
4. Stratified transitional	4.	4.
5.	5. Surface of lining of trachea	5.
6.	6.	6. Secretion; absorption
Connective		
1.	1. Between other tissues and organs	1.
2. Adipose	2.	2.
3.	3.	3. Flexible but strong connection
4.	4. Skeleton	4.
5.	5. Part of nasal septum, larynx, rings in trachea and bronchi, disks between vertebrae, external ear	5.
6.	6.	6. Transportation
7. Hemopoietic tissue	7.	7.
Muscle		
1.	1. Muscles that attach to bones, eyeball muscles, upper third of esophagus	1.
2. Cardiac	2.	
3.	3. Walls of digestive, respiratory, and genitourinary tracts; walls of blood and large lymphatic vessels; ducts of glands; intrinsic eye muscles; arrector muscles of hair	3.
Nervous		
1. Nerve cells	1. Brain and spinal cord, nerves	1.

Unscramble the words

43. Translation
44. Interphase
45. Gene
46. Osmosis
47. Diffusion
48. Tissues

Applying what you know

49.

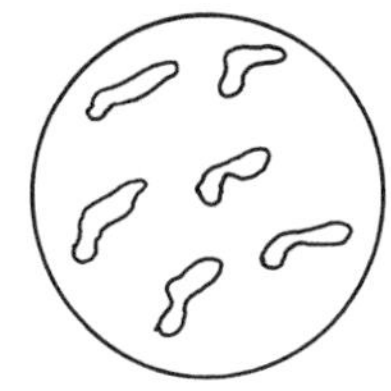

50. Diffusion
51. Absorption of oxygen into Ms. Bence's blood.
52. Merrily may have exceeded the 18–24% desirable body fat composition. Fitness depends more on the percentage and ratio of specific tissue types than the overall amount of tissue present.

53. WORD FIND

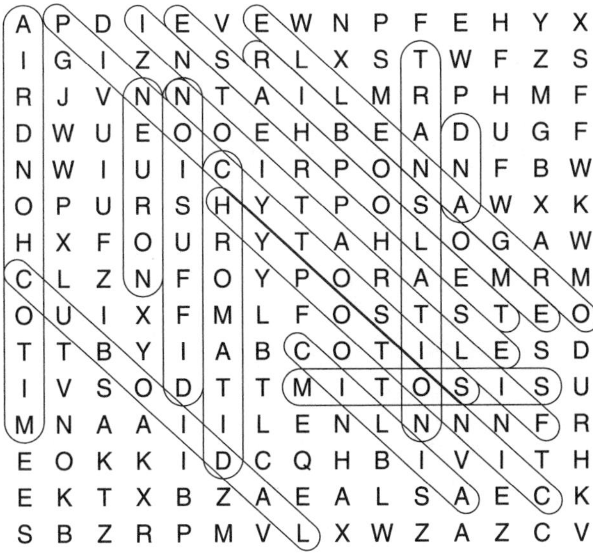

Crossword

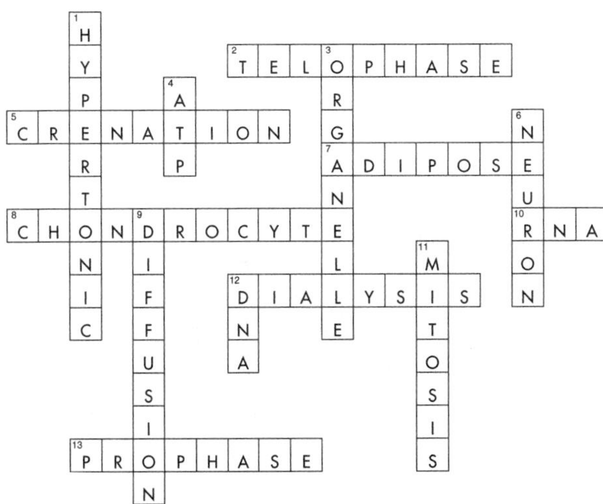

Check your knowledge

Multiple choice

1. A, p. 44
2. B, p. 44
3. B, p. 45
4. A, p. 48
5. C, p. 52
6. A, p. 54
7. D, p. 55
8. B, p. 57
9. C, p. 68
10. D, p. 61

Matching

11. F, p. 45
12. G, p. 48
13. J, p. 48
14. C, p. 51
15. A, p. 53
16. B, p. 54
17. I, p. 57
18. H, p. 59
19. D, p. 59
20. E, p. 67

Cell structure

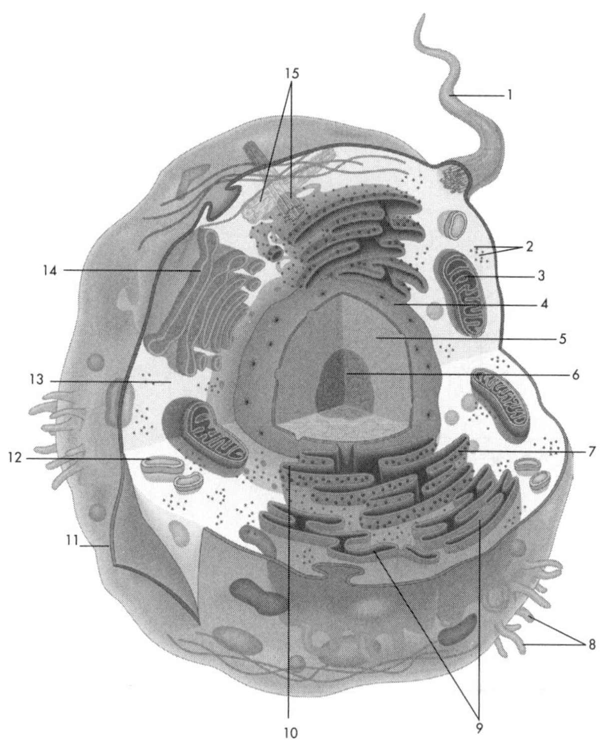

1. Flagellum
2. Free ribosomes
3. Mitochondrion
4. Nuclear envelope
5. Nucleus
6. Nucleolus
7. Ribosomes
8. Cilia
9. Smooth endoplasmic reticulum
10. Rough endoplasmic reticulum
11. Plasma membrane
12. Lysosome
13. Cytoplasm
14. Golgi apparatus
15. Centrioles

Mitosis

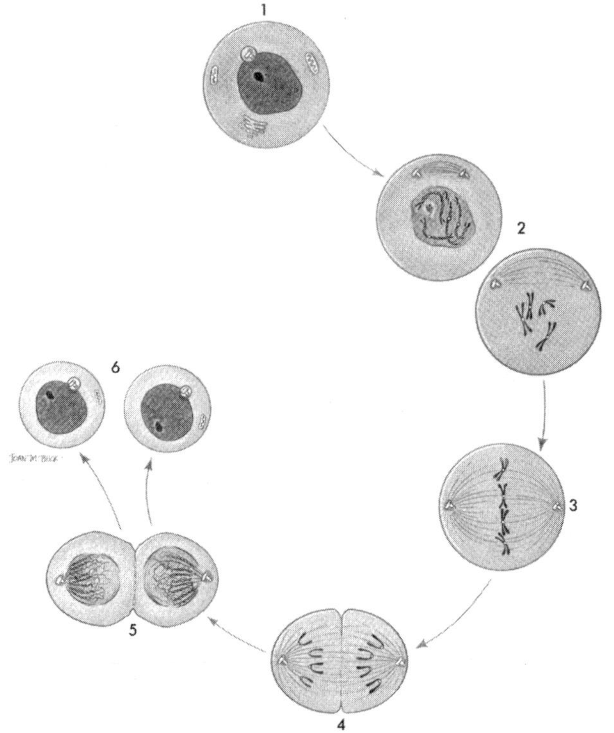

1. Interphase
2. Prophase
3. Metaphase
4. Anaphase
5. Telophase
6. Daughter cells (interphase)

Tissues

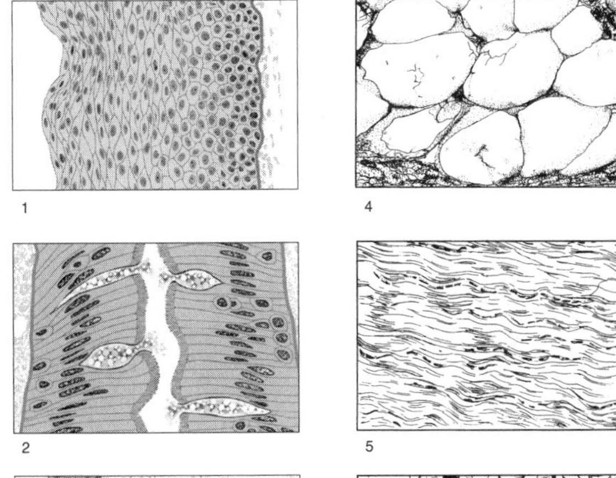

1. Stratified squamous epithelium
2. Simple columnar epithelium
3. Stratified transitional epithelium
4. Adipose tissue
5. Dense fibrous connective tissue
6. Bone tissue

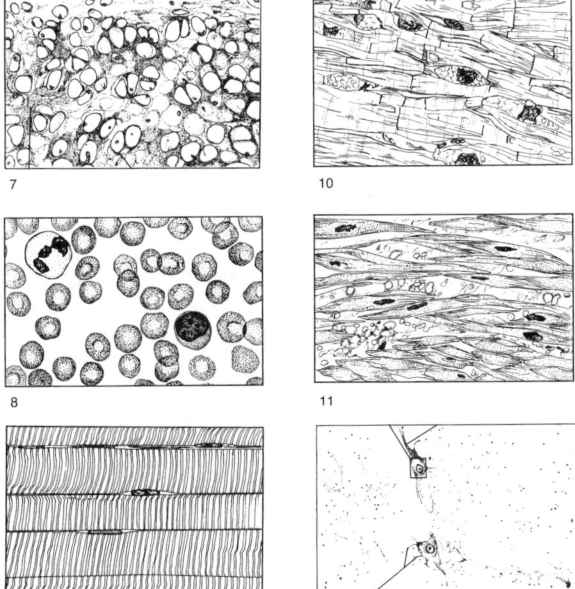

7. Cartilage
8. Blood
9. Skeletal muscle
10. Cardiac muscle
11. Smooth muscle
12. Nervous tissue

CHAPTER 4
ORGAN SYSTEMS OF THE BODY

Matching

Group A

1. A, p. 80
2. E, p. 83
3. D, p. 83
4. B, p. 83
5. C, p. 84

Group B

6. F, p. 85
7. E, p. 86
8. B, p. 88
9. A, p. 88
10. C, p. 86
11. D, p. 90

Circle the one that does not belong

12. Mouth (the others refer to the respiratory system)
13. Rectum (the others refer to the reproductive system)
14. Pancreas (the others refer to the circulatory system)
15. Pineal (the others refer to the urinary system)
16. Joints (the others refer to the muscular system)
17. Pituitary (the others refer to the nervous system)
18. Tendons (the others refer to the skeletal system)
19. Appendix (the others refer to the endocrine system)
20. Thymus (the others refer to the integumentary system)
21. Trachea (the others refer to the digestive system)
22. Liver (the others refer to the lymphatic system)

Fill in the missing areas

SYSTEM	ORGANS	FUNCTIONS
		23. Protection, regulation of body temperature, synthesis of chemicals and hormones, serves as a sense organ
	24. Bones, joints	
		25. Movement, maintains body posture, produces heat
26. Nervous		
	27. Pituitary, thymus, pineal, adrenal, hypothalamus, thyroid, pancreas, parathyroid, ovaries, testes	
		28. Transportation, immunity
	29. Lymph nodes, lymph vessels, thymus, spleen, tonsils	
30. Urinary		
	31. Mouth, pharynx, esophagus, stomach, small and large intestine, rectum, anal canal, teeth, salivary glands, tongue, liver, gallbladder, pancreas, appendix	
32. Respiratory		
	33. a. Gonads—testes and ovaries	
	b. Accessory organs, ducts, and glands (p. 90) Supporting structures (p. 90)	

Unscramble the words

34. Heart
35. Pineal
36. Nerve
37. Esophagus
38. Nervous

Applying what you know

39. Endocrinology (endocrine system); gynecology (reproductive system)
40. The skin protects the underlying tissue against invasion by harmful bacteria. With a large percentage of Brian's skin destroyed, he was vulnerable to bacteria, and so he was placed in the cleanest environment possible—isolation. Jenny is required to wear special attire so that the risk of her bringing bacteria to the patient is reduced.

41.

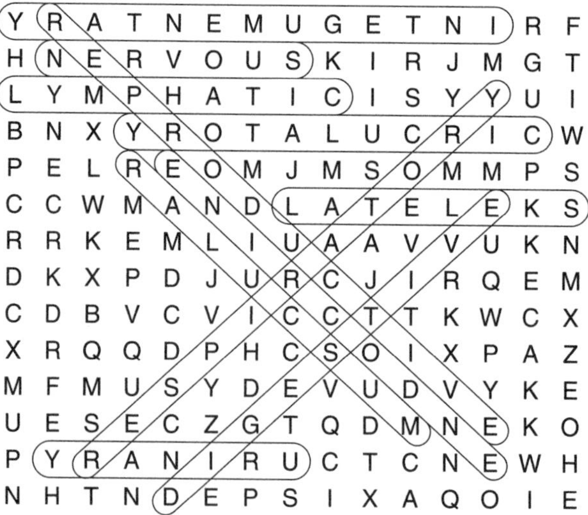

Crossword

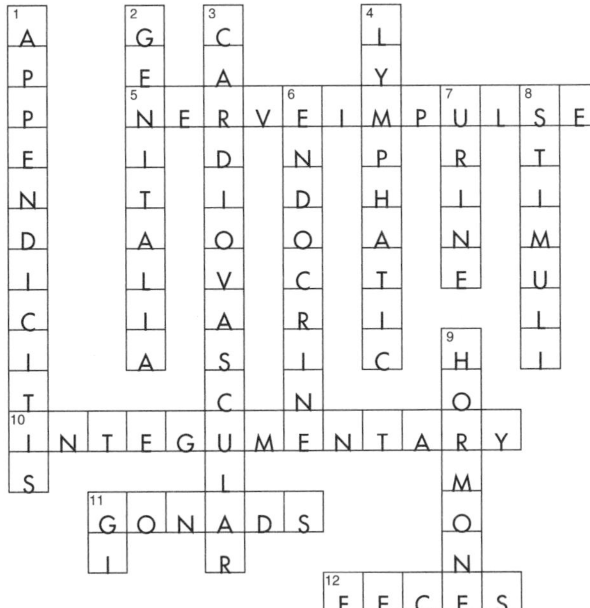

Check your knowledge

Multiple choice

1. D, p. 84
2. C, p. 86
3. C, p. 90
4. B, p. 80
5. D, p. 83
6. A, p. 80
7. B, p. 88
8. A, p. 84
9. A, p. 84
10. C, p. 79

Matching

11. C, p. 80
12. D, p. 85
13. H, p. 86
14. G, p. 90
15. B, p. 88
16. F, p. 88
17. I, p. 90
18. E, p. 86
19. J, p. 84
20. A, p. 84

CHAPTER 5 THE INTEGUMENTARY SYSTEM AND BODY MEMBRANES

Select the best answer

1. B, p. 100
2. D, p. 102
3. C, p. 100
4. A, p. 100
5. B, p. 100
6. D, p. 102
7. C, p. 100
8. C, p. 100

Matching

Group A

9. D, p. 102
10. A, p. 102
11. B, p. 102
12. C, p. 106
13. E, p. 102

Group B

14. A, p. 103
15. D, p. 104
16. E, p. 103
17. C, p. 105
18. B, p. 105

Select the correct term

19. A, p. 102
20. B, p. 106
21. B, p. 105
22. A, p. 105
23. A, p. 103
24. B, p. 100
25. B, p. 106
26. B, p. 109
27. B, p. 108
28. A, p. 104 (Fig. 5-3)

Fill in the blanks

29. Protection, temperature regulation, and sense organ activity, p. 110
30. Melanin, p. 104
31. Lanugo, p. 106
32. Hair papillae, p. 106
33. Lunula, p. 108
34. Arrector pili, p. 107
35. Light touch, p. 108
36. Eccrine, p. 108
37. Apocrine, p. 109
38. Sebum, p. 109

Circle the correct answer

39. Will not, p. 112
40. Will, p. 112
41. Will not, p. 113
42. 11, p. 112
43. Third, p. 112

Unscramble the words

44. Epidermis
45. Keratin
46. Hair
47. Lanugo
48. Dehydration
49. Third degree

Applying what you know

50. 46
51. Pleurisy
52. Fingerprints

53.

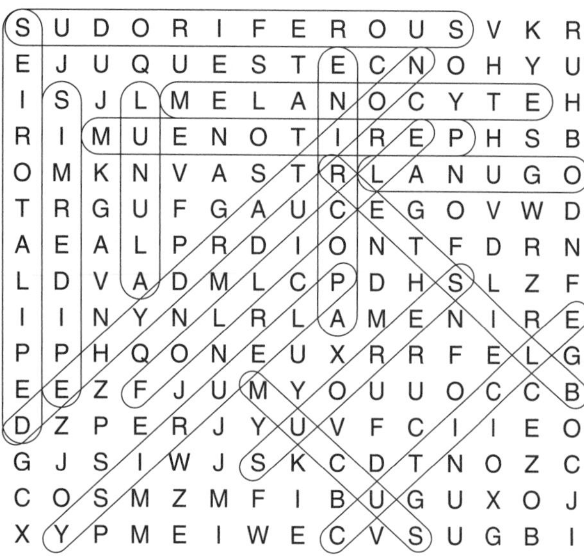

Crossword

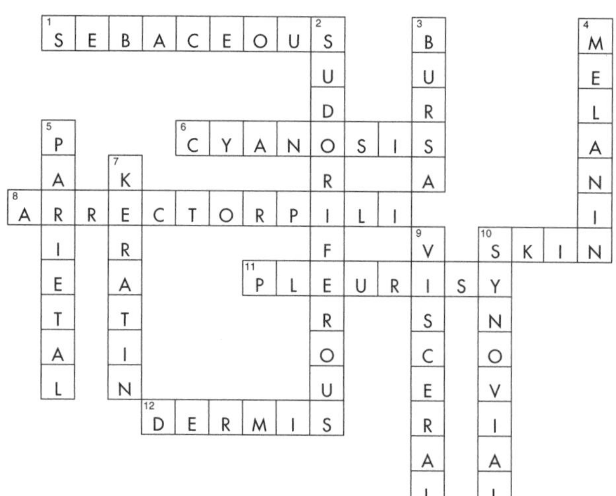

Check your knowledge

Multiple choice

1. A, p. 100
2. B, p. 100
3. A, p. 105
4. D, p. 103
5. B, p. 105
6. D, p. 106
7. B, p. 108
8. B, p. 108
9. C, p. 108
10. B, p. 109

Matching

11. C, p. 100
12. D, p. 100
13. B, p. 100
14. G, p. 100
15. I, p. 102
16. H, p. 106
17. J, p. 106
18. E, p. 107
19. A, p. 108
20. F, p. 108

Completion

21. H, p. 99
22. A, p. 103
23. B, p. 100
24. F, p. 102
25. I, p. 112
26. E, p. 112
27. G, p. 112
28. D, p. 112
29. J, p. 109
30. C, p. 108

Longitudinal section of the skin

1. Opening of sweat ducts
2. Epidermis
3. Dermis
4. Subcutaneous fatty tissue (hypodermis)
5. Sweat gland
6. Arrector pili muscle
7. Pacinian corpuscle
8. Cutaneous nerve
9. Papilla of hair
10. Hair follicle
11. Sebaceous (oil) gland
12. Meissner's corpuscle
13. Dermal papilla
14. Stratum germinativum
15. Stratum corneum
16. Hair shaft

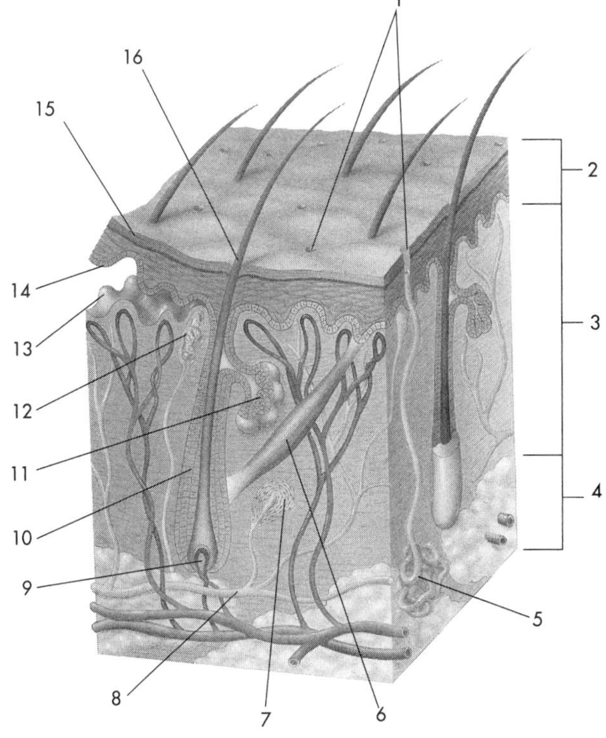

"Rule of Nines" for estimating skin surface burned

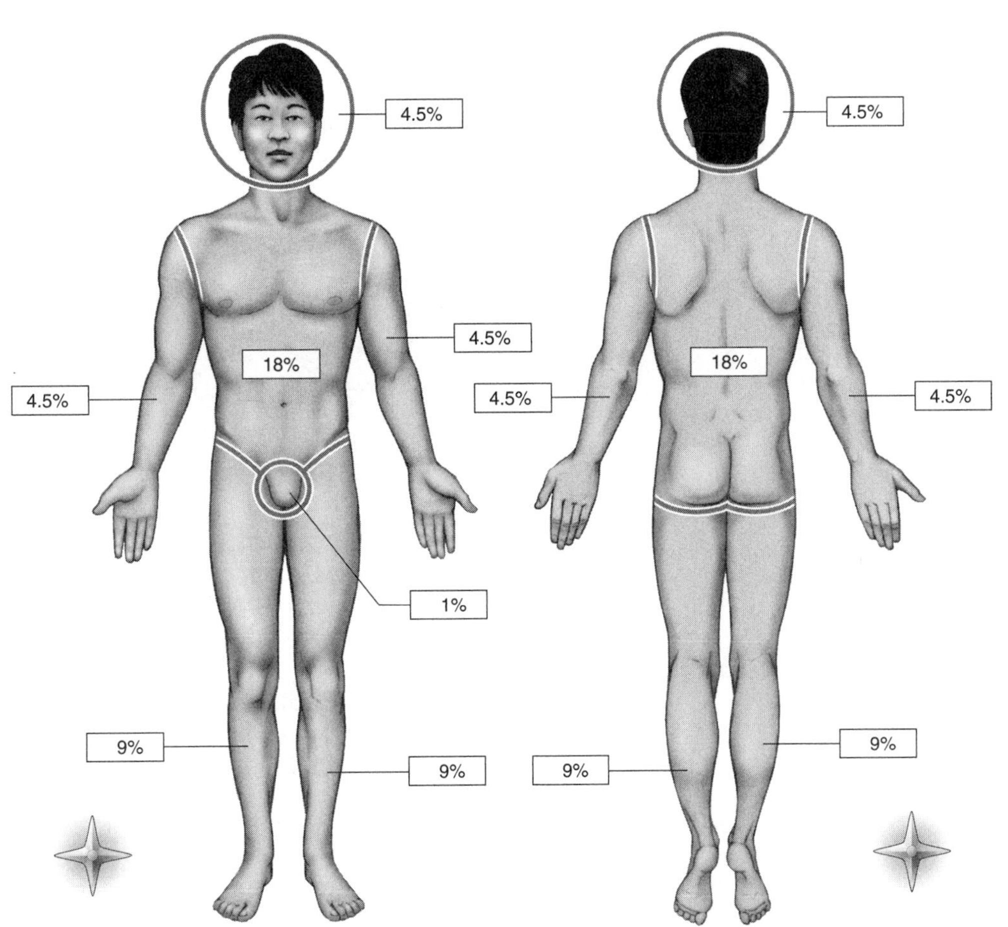

CHAPTER 6 THE SKELETAL SYSTEM

Fill in the blanks

1. 4, p. 122
2. Medullary cavity, p. 122
3. Articular cartilage p. 122
4. Endosteum, p. 122
5. Hemopoiesis, p. 122
6. Red bone marrow, p. 122
7. Periosteum, p. 122
8. Elderly white females, p. 127
9. Calcium, p. 122
10. Move, p. 122

Matching

Group A

11. D, p. 123
12. B, p. 123
13. E, p. 123
14. A, p. 122
15. C, p. 123

Group B

16. D, p. 123
17. A, p. 123
18. E, p. 123
19. B, p. 123
20. C, p. 123

True or false

21. T
22. Epiphyses, not diaphyses, p. 122
23. Osteoblasts, not osteoclasts, p. 125
24. T
25. Increase, not decrease, p. 125
26. Juvenile, not adult, p. 125
27. Diaphysis, not articulation, p. 125
28. T
29. Ceases, not begins, p. 125
30. T

Multiple choice

31. A, p. 127
32. D, p. 131
33. A, p. 134
34. D, p. 135
35. C, p. 136
36. C, p. 139
37. D, p. 136
38. D, p. 139
39. A, p. 139
40. B, p. 131
41. A, p. 134
42. B, p. 138
43. B, p. 135
44. B, p. 136
45. C, p. 139
46. A, p. 139
47. D, p. 131
48. C, p. 134
49. C, p. 131

Circle the one that does not belong

50. Coxal bone (all others refer to the spine)
51. Axial (all others refer to the appendicular skeleton)
52. Maxilla (all others refer to the cranial bones)
53. Ribs (all others refer to the shoulder girdle)
54. Vomer (all others refer to the bones of the middle ear)
55. Ulna (all others refer to the coxal bone)
56. Ethmoid (all others refer to the hand and wrist)
57. Nasal (all others refer to cranial bones)
58. Anvil (all others refer to the cervical vertebra)

Choose the correct term

59. A, p. 139
60. B, p. 139
61. B, p. 127
62. A, p. 139
63. B, p. 139

Matching

64. C, p. 131
65. G, p. 135
66. J, L, M, and K, p. 141
67. N, p. 141
68. I, p. 138
69. A, p. 131
70. P, p. 141
71. D, B, p. 131
72. F, p. 131
73. H, Q, p. 138
74. O, T, p. 141
75. R, p. 131
76. S, E, p. 131

Circle the correct answer

77. Diarthroses, p. 143
78. Synarthrotic, p. 142
79. Diarthrotic, p. 143
80. Ligaments, p. 144
81. Articular cartilage, p. 144
82. Least movable, p. 145
83. Largest, p. 147
84. 2, p. 144
85. Mobility, p. 144
86. Pivot, p. 144

Unscramble the words

87. Vertebrae
88. Pubis
89. Scapula
90. Mandible
91. Phalanges
92. Pelvic girdle

Applying what you know

93. The bones are responsible for the majority of our blood cell formation. The disease condition of the bones might be inhibiting the production of blood cells for Mrs. Perine.
94. Epiphyseal cartilage is present only while a child is still growing. It becomes bone in adulthood. It is particularly vulnerable to fractures in childhood and preadolescence.
95. Osteoporosis

96.

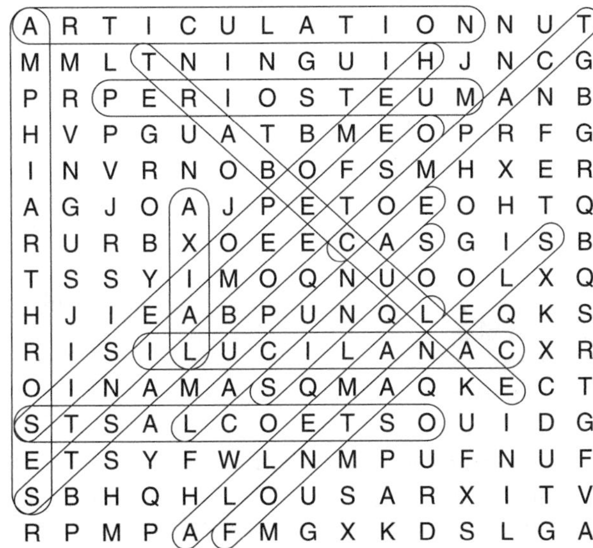

Crossword

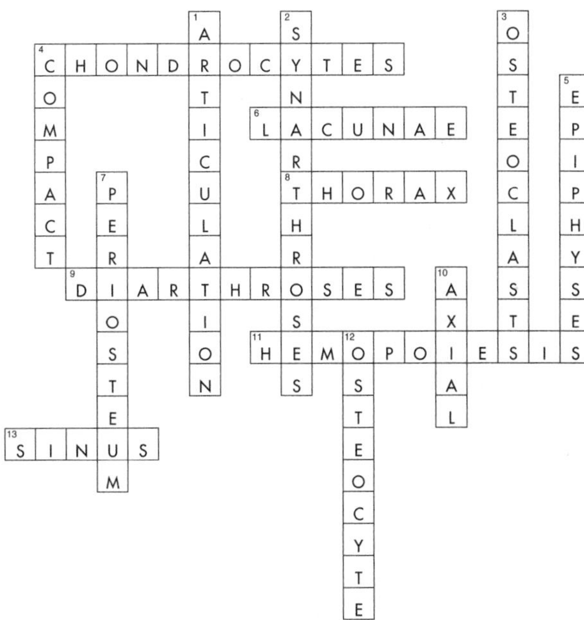

Check your knowledge

Multiple choice

1. A, p. 122
2. C, p. 122
3. A, p. 122
4. C, p. 127
5. C, pp. 136 and 139
6. D, p. 125
7. C, p. 130
8. C, p. 135
9. D, p. 139 and Table 6-6
10. A, p. 143

Matching

11. G, p. 142
12. B, p. 122
13. I, p. 123
14. J, p. 131
15. E, p. 135
16. H, p. 131
17. A, p. 138
18. C, p. 142
19. F, p. 144
20. D, p. 145

Longitudinal section of long bone

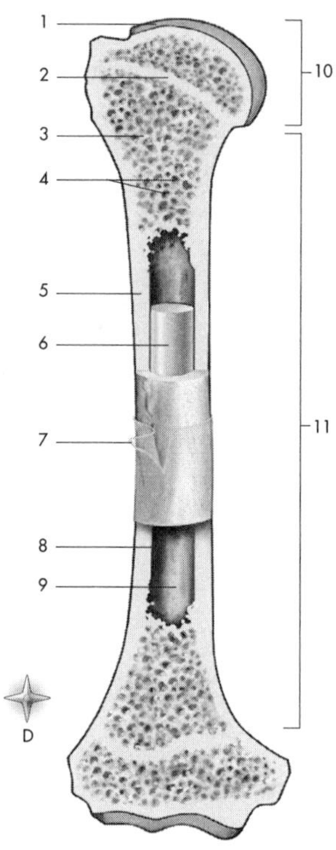

1. Articular cartilage
2. Epiphyseal line
3. Spongy bone
4. Red marrow cavities
5. Compact bone
6. Yellow marrow
7. Periosteum
8. Endosteum
9. Medullary cavity
10. Epiphysis
11. Diaphysis

Anterior view of skeleton

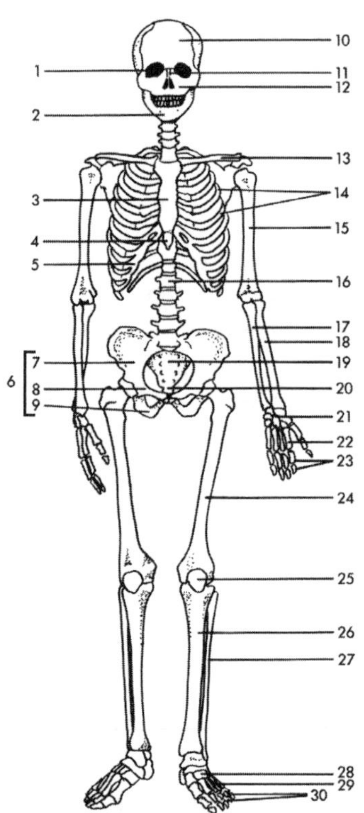

1. Orbit
2. Mandible
3. Sternum
4. Xiphoid process
5. Costal cartilage
6. Coxal (hip) bone
7. Ilium
8. Pubis
9. Ischium
10. Frontal
11. Nasal
12. Maxilla
13. Clavicle
14. Ribs
15. Humerus
16. Vertebral column
17. Ulna
18. Radius
19. Sacrum
20. Coccyx
21. Carpals
22. Metacarpals
23. Phalanges
24. Femur
25. Patella
26. Tibia
27. Fibula
28. Tarsals
29. Metatarsals
30. Phalanges

Posterior view of skeleton

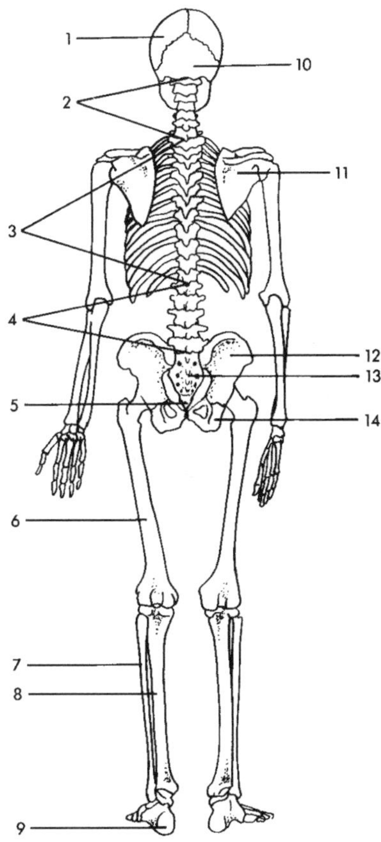

1. Parietal
2. Cervical vertebrae
3. Thoracic vertebrae
4. Lumbar vertebrae
5. Coccyx
6. Femur
7. Fibula
8. Tibia
9. Calcaneus
10. Occipital
11. Scapula
12. Ilium
13. Sacrum
14. Ischium

Skull viewed from the right side

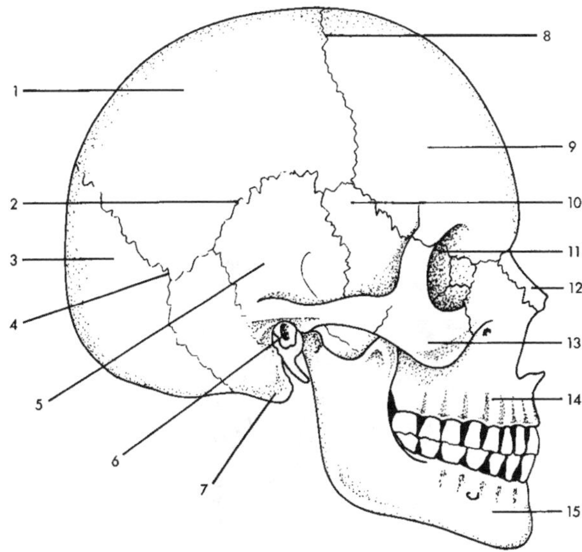

1. Parietal bone
2. Squamous suture
3. Occipital bone
4. Lambdoidal suture
5. Temporal bone
6. External auditory canal
7. Mastoid process
8. Coronal suture
9. Frontal bone
10. Sphenoid bone
11. Ethmoid bone
12. Nasal bone
13. Zygomatic bone
14. Maxilla
15. Mandible

Skull viewed from the front

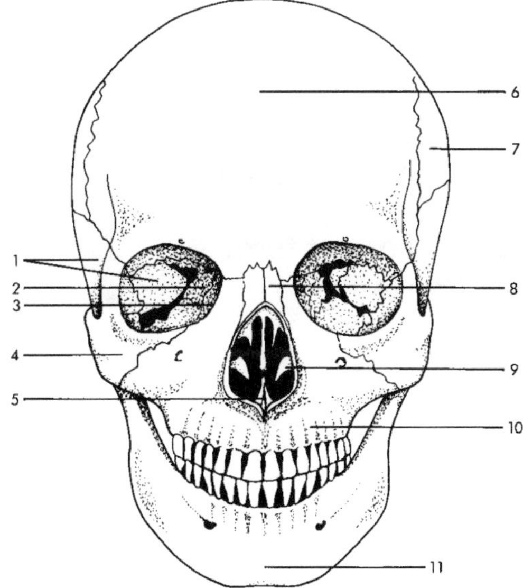

1. Sphenoid bone
2. Ethmoid bone
3. Lacrimal bone
4. Zygomatic bone
5. Vomer
6. Frontal bone
7. Parietal bone
8. Nasal bone
9. Inferior concha
10. Maxilla
11. Mandible

Structure of a diarthrotic joint

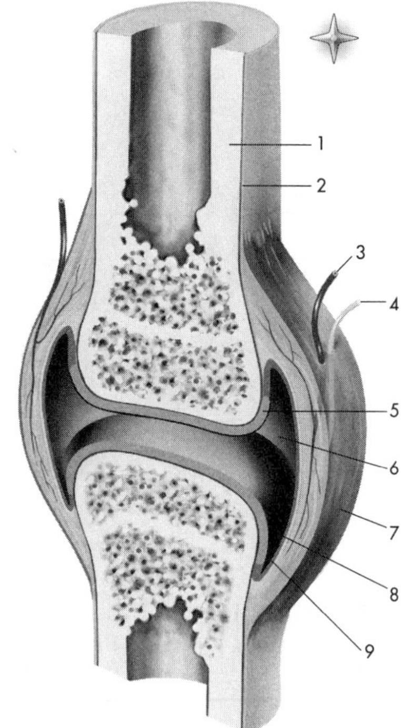

1. Bone
2. Periosteum
3. Blood vessel
4. Nerve
5. Articular cartilage
6. Joint cavity
7. Joint capsule
8. Articular cartilage
9. Synovial membrane

CHAPTER 7
THE MUSCULAR SYSTEM

Select the correct term

1. A, p. 156 and B, p. 156
2. B, p. 156
3. C, p. 157
4. C, p. 156
5. A, p. 156
6. B, p. 157
7. C and B, p. 156
8. A, p. 155
9. C, p. 156
10. C, p. 157

Matching

Group A

11. D, p. 157
12. B, p. 157
13. A, p. 157
14. E, p. 157
15. C, p. 157

Group B

16. E, p. 157
17. C, p. 157
18. B, p. 157
19. A, p. 157
20. D, p. 157

Fill in the blanks

21. Pulling, p. 159
22. Insertion, p. 159
23. Insertion, origin, p. 159
24. Prime mover, p. 159
25. Antagonists, p. 159
26. Synergist, p. 159
27. Tonic contraction, p. 160
28. Muscle tone, p. 160
29. Hypothermia, p. 160
30. ATP, p. 160

True or false

31. Neuromuscular junction, p. 161
32. T
33. T
34. Oxygen debt, p. 160
35. "All or none," p. 162
36. Lactic acid, p. 160
37. T
38. T
39. Skeletal muscle, p. 160
40. T

Circle the correct answer

41. A, p. 162
42. B, p. 162
43. B, p. 162
44. C, p. 164
45. D, p. 164
46. A, p. 162
47. B, p. 162
48. C, p. 162
49. B, p. 164
50. D, p. 164

Select the best choice or choices

51. C, p. 168
52. F, p. 169, A and D, p. 175
53. F, p. 169, and B, p. 175
54. A, p. 168
55. C, p. 175
56. B, p. 175, and F, p. 169
57. A, p. 175
58. A and D, pp. 168 and 175
59. B, p. 168

60. B, p. 168
61. A, p. 168, and E, p. 168
62. B, p. 168
63. D, p. 168

Circle the correct answer

64. A, p. 172
65. D, p. 173
66. C, p. 173
67. A, p. 173
68. D, p. 173
69. C, p. 173

Applying what you know

70. Bursitis
71. Deltoid area
72. Tendon

73.

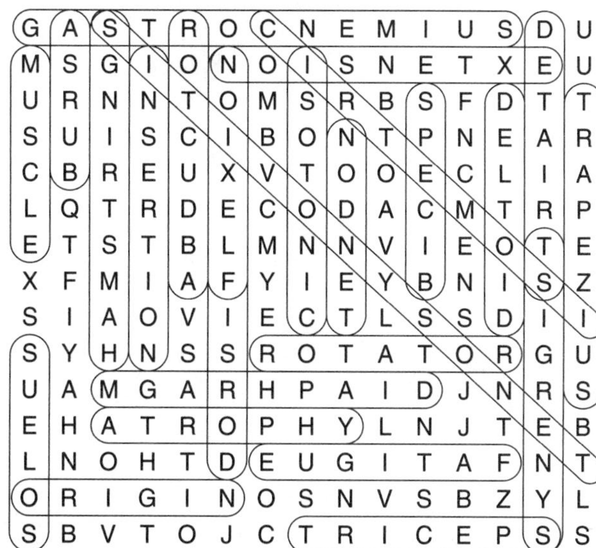

Crossword

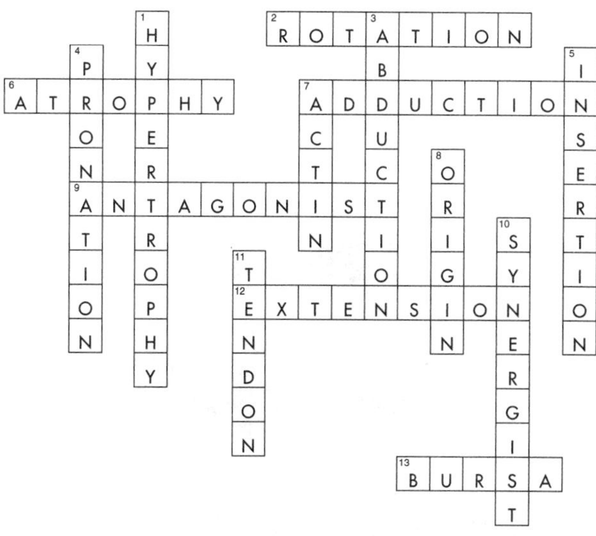

Check your knowledge

Multiple choice

1. D, p. 164
2. A, p. 164
3. C, p. 162
4. B, p. 161
5. A, p. 159
6. B, p. 159
7. D, p. 160
8. A, p. 157
9. A, p. 156
10. C, p. 171

True or false

11. T
12. T
13. F, myosin, p. 157
14. F, posterior, p. 170
15. T
16. T
17. T
18. F, flexion, p. 172
19. T
20. F, smiling, p. 165

Muscles—anterior view

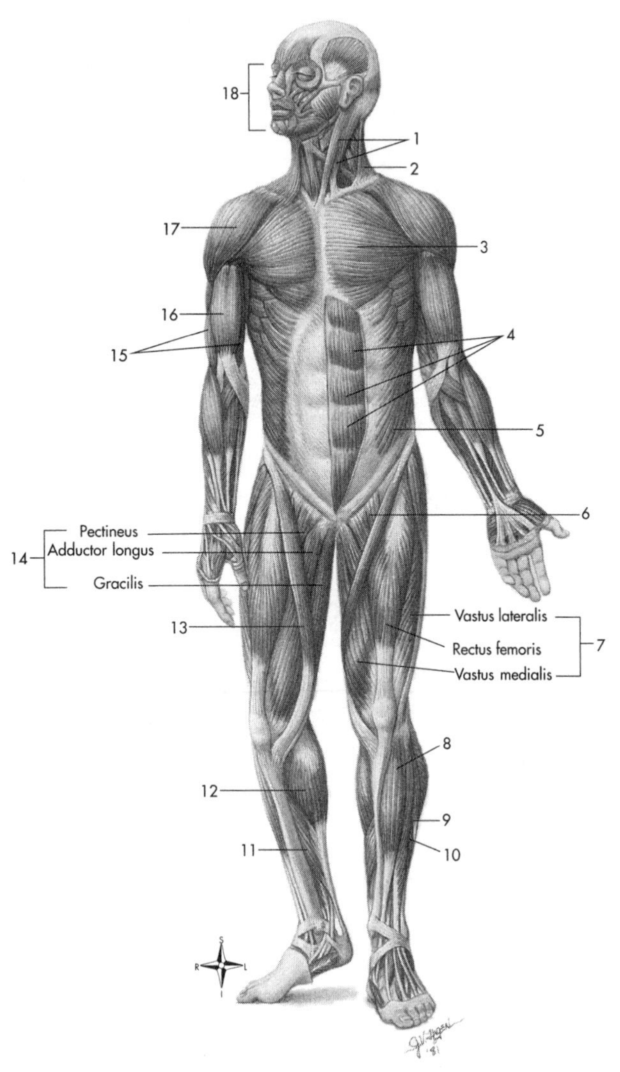

1. Sternocleidomastoid
2. Trapezius
3. Pectoralis major
4. Rectus abdominis
5. External abdominal oblique
6. Iliopsoas
7. Quadriceps group
8. Tibialis anterior
9. Peroneus longus
10. Peroneus brevis
11. Soleus
12. Gastrocnemius
13. Sartorius
14. Adductor group
15. Brachialis
16. Biceps brachii
17. Deltoid
18. Facial muscles

Muscles—posterior view

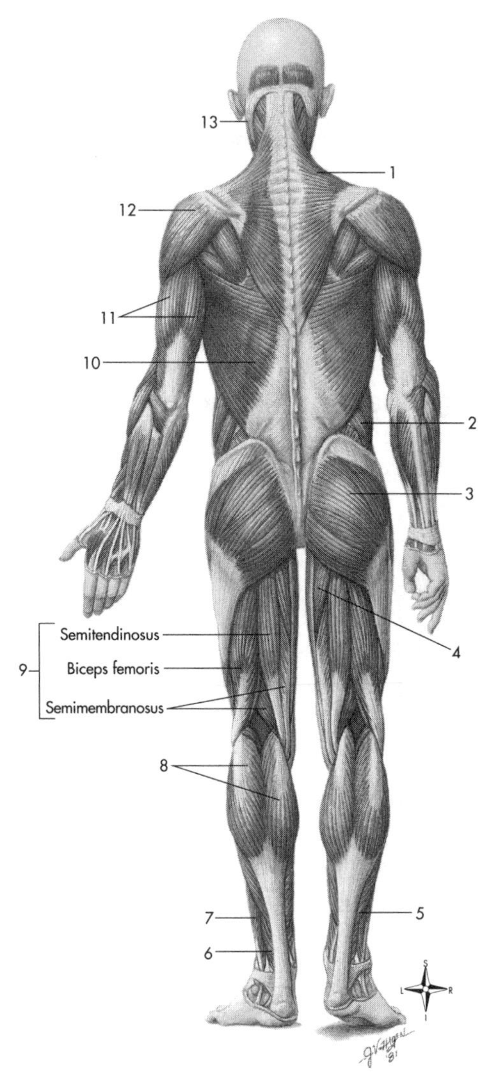

1. Trapezius
2. External abdominal oblique
3. Gluteus maximus
4. Adductor magnus
5. Soleus
6. Peroneus brevis
7. Peroneus longus
8. Gastrocnemius
9. Hamstring group
10. Latissimus dorsi
11. Triceps brachii
12. Deltoid
13. Sternocleidomastoid

CHAPTER 8
THE NERVOUS SYSTEM

Matching

Group A
1. B, p. 186
2. C, p. 186
3. D, p. 186
4. A, p. 187

Group B
5. B, p. 187
6. D, p. 187
7. C, p. 187
8. A, p. 187
9. F, p. 190
10. E, p. 190

Select the correct term
11. A, p. 187
12. B, p. 187
13. B, p. 187
14. A, p. 187
15. A, p. 187
16. B, p. 189
17. B, p. 189
18. A, p. 187
19. B, p. 192
20. A, p. 187

Fill in the blanks
21. Two-neuron arc, p. 191
22. Sensory, interneurons, and motor neurons, p. 192
23. Receptors, p. 191
24. Synapse, p. 191
25. Reflex, p. 192
26. Withdrawal reflex, p. 192
27. Ganglion, p. 191
28. Interneurons, p. 192
29. "Knee jerk," p. 191
30. Gray matter, p. 193

Circle the correct answer
31. Do not, p. 193
32. Increases, p. 193
33. Excess, p. 193
34. Postsynaptic, p. 193
35. Presynaptic, p. 193
36. Neurotransmitter, p. 195
37. Communicate, p. 195
38. Specifically, p. 195
39. Sleep, p. 196
40. Pain, p. 196

Circle the correct answer
41. E, p. 196
42. D, p. 197
43. A, p. 197
44. E, p. 197
45. E, p. 199
46. D, p. 199
47. B, p. 199
48. E, p. 201
49. B, p. 201
50. D, p. 201
51. D, p. 199
52. B, p. 201
53. A, p. 201
54. D, p. 202
55. C, p. 199

True or false
56. 17 to 18 inches, p. 202
57. Bottom of the first lumbar vertebra, p. 202
58. Lumbar punctures, p. 208
59. Spinal tracts, p. 203
60. T
61. One general function, p. 203
62. Anesthesia, p. 205

Circle the one that does not belong
63. Ventricles (all others refer to meninges)
64. CSF (all others refer to the arachnoid)
65. Pia mater (all others refer to the cerebrospinal fluid)
66. Choroid plexus (all others refer to the dura mater)
67. Brain tumor (all others refer to a lumbar puncture)

68. Fill in the missing areas on the chart below.

NERVE		CONDUCT IMPULSES	FUNCTION
I	Olfactory		
II			Vision
III		From brain to eye muscles	
IV	Trochlear		
V			Sensations of face, scalp, and teeth, chewing movements
VI		From brain to external eye muscles	
VII		Sense of taste; contractions of muscles of facial expression	
VIII	Vestibulocochlear		
IX		From throat and taste buds of tongue to brain; also from brain to throat muscles and salivary glands	
X	Vagus		
XI			Shoulder movements; turning movements of head
XII	Hypoglossal		

Select the correct term

69. A, p. 208
70. B, p. 210
71. A, p. 208
72. B, p. 216
73. B, p. 208
74. A, p. 208
75. B, p. 208
76. B, p. 209

Matching

77. D, p. 210
78. E, p. 211
79. F, p. 211
80. B, p. 211
81. A, p. 211
82. C, p. 210

Circle the correct answer

83. C, p. 213
84. B, p. 213
85. B, p. 215
86. D, p. 213
87. A, p. 215
88. A, p. 215

Select the correct term

89. B, p. 214
90. A, p. 214
91. A, p. 214
92. B, p. 214
93. A, p. 214
94. B, p. 214
95. A, p. 214
96. A, p. 214
97. B, p. 214
98. B, p. 214

Fill in the blanks

99. Acetylcholine, p. 215
100. Adrenergic fibers, p. 216
101. Cholinergic fibers, p. 215
102. Homeostasis, p. 216
103. Heart rate, p. 216
104. Decreased, p. 216

Unscramble the words

105. Neurons
106. Synapse
107. Autonomic
108. Smooth muscle
109. Sympathetic

Applying what you know

110. Right
111. Hydrocephalus
112. Sympathetic
113. Parasympathetic

114. Sympathetic; No, the digestive process is not active during sympathetic control. Bill may experience nausea, vomiting, or discomfort because of this factor. See p. 214.

115.

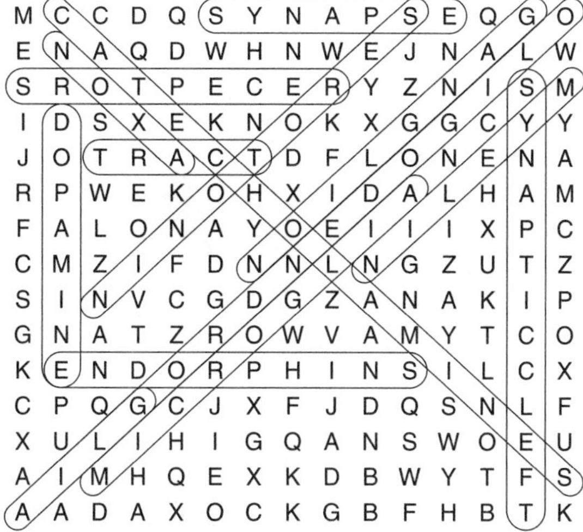

Crossword

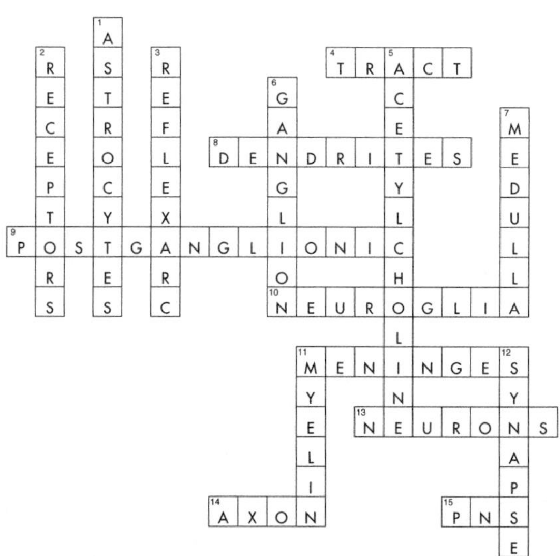

Check your knowledge

Multiple choice

1. D, p. 187
2. B, p. 187
3. A, p. 189
4. B, p. 191
5. A, p. 191
6. D, p. 193
7. D, p. 196
8. C, p. 199
9. C, p. 205
10. D, p. 210

Matching

11. C, p. 192
12. A, p. 199
13. J, p. 201
14. H, p. 206
15. B, p. 210
16. I, p. 208
17. F, p. 211
18. E, p. 215
19. D, p. 215
20. G, p. 202

Neuron

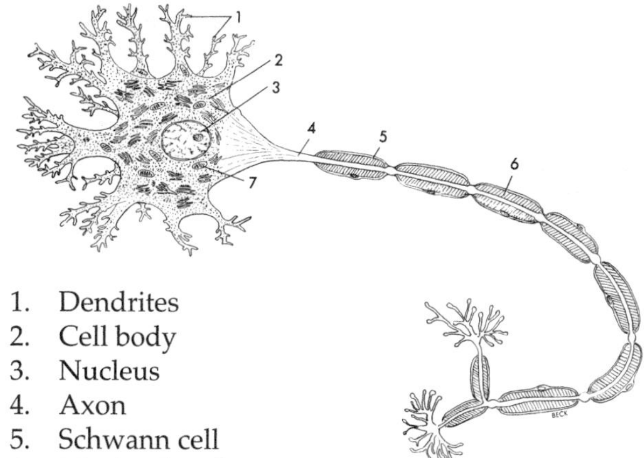

1. Dendrites
2. Cell body
3. Nucleus
4. Axon
5. Schwann cell
6. Myelin sheath
7. Mitochondrion

Cranial nerves

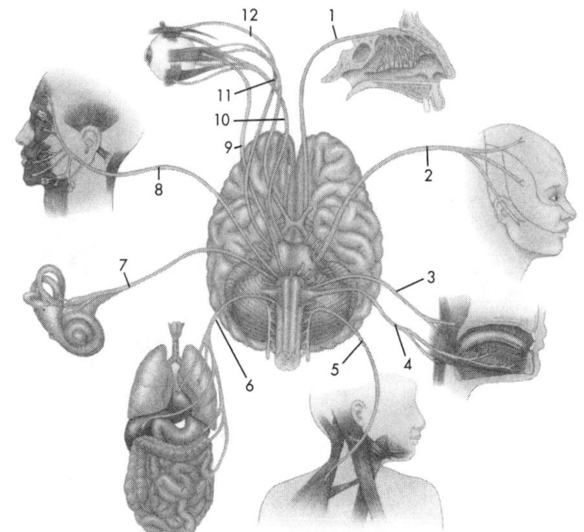

1. Olfactory nerve
2. Trigeminal nerve
3. Glossopharyngeal nerve
4. Hypoglossal nerve
5. Accessory nerve
6. Vagus nerve
7. Vestibulocochlear nerve
8. Facial nerve
9. Abducens nerve
10. Oculomotor nerve
11. Optic nerve
12. Trochlear nerve

Neural pathway involved in the patellar reflex

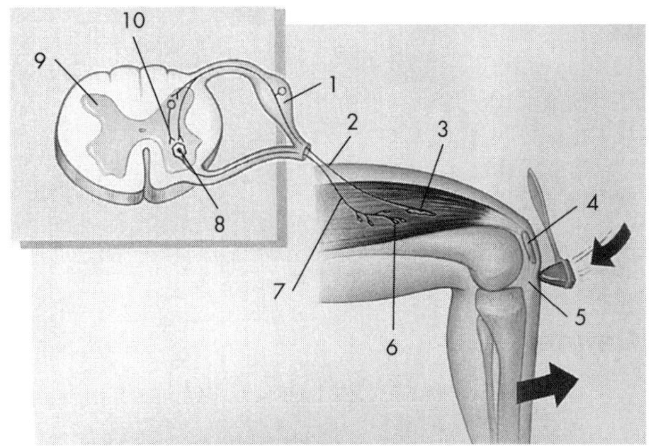

1. Dorsal root ganglion
2. Sensory neuron
3. Stretch receptor
4. Patella
5. Patellar tendon
6. Quadriceps muscle
7. Motor neuron
8. Monosynaptic synapse
9. Gray matter
10. Interneuron

Sagittal section of the central nervous system

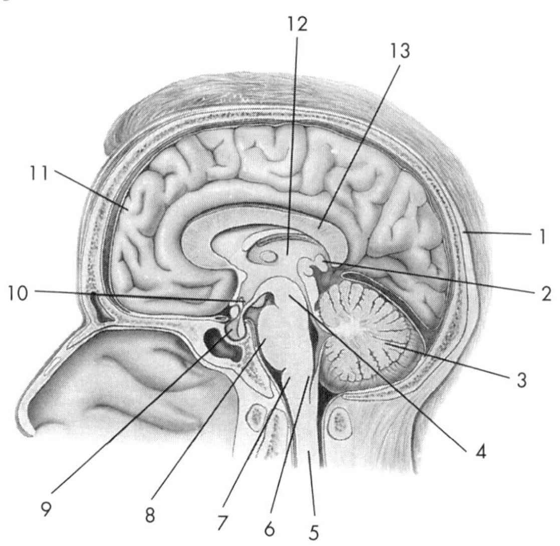

1. Skull
2. Pineal gland
3. Cerebellum
4. Midbrain
5. Spinal cord
6. Medulla
7. Reticular formation
8. Pons
9. Pituitary gland
10. Hypothalamus
11. Cerebral cortex
12. Thalamus
13. Corpus callosum

The cerebrum

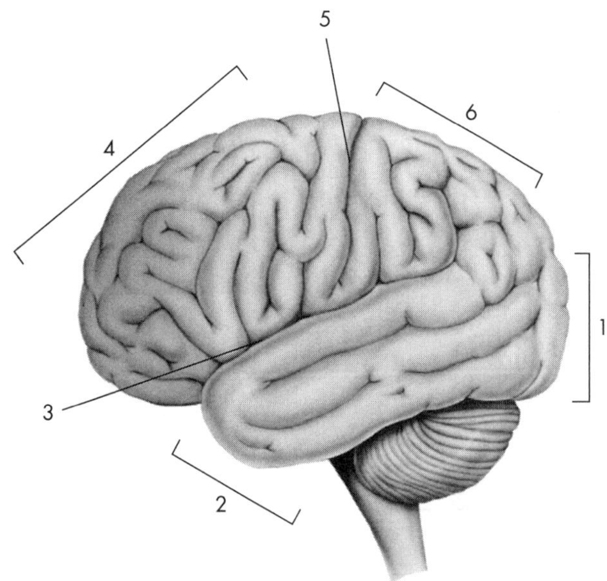

1. Occipital lobe
2. Temporal lobe
3. Lateral fissure
4. Frontal lobe
5. Central sulcus
6. Parietal lobe

Autonomic conduction paths

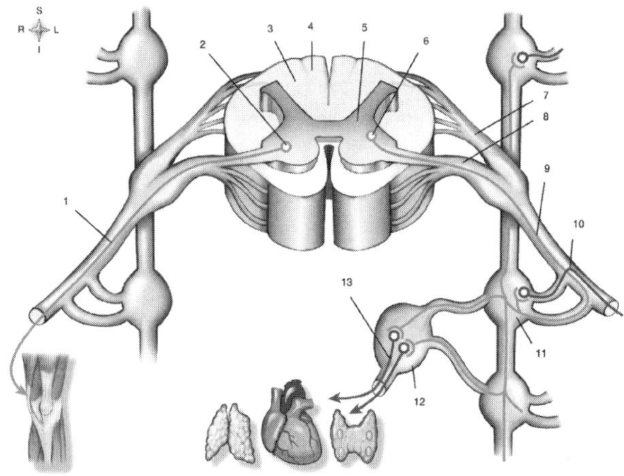

1. Axon of somatic motor neuron
2. Cell body of somatic motor neuron
3. White matter
4. Spinal cord
5. Gray matter
6. Cell body of preganglionic neuron
7. Dorsal root
8. Ventral root
9. Axon of preganglionic sympathetic neuron
10. Axon of postganglionic neuron
11. Sympathetic ganglion
12. Collateral ganglion
13. Axon of postganglionic sympathetic neuron

CHAPTER 9
SENSE ORGANS

Matching
1. D, p. 230
2. B, p. 228
3. A, p. 230
4. E, p. 229
5. C, p. 230

Circle the correct answer
6. C, p. 231
7. E, p. 231
8. B, p. 231
9. C, p. 231
10. E, p. 231
11. D, p. 233
12. A, p. 233
13. B, p. 233
14. C, p. 235
15. B, p. 235
16. D, p. 234
17. A, p. 235
18. D, p. 236

Select the correct term
19. B, p. 238
20. C, p. 239
21. B, p. 238
22. A, p. 238
23. C, p. 239
24. A, p. 238
25. C, p. 239
26. B, p. 238
27. B, p. 238
28. C, p. 239

Fill in the blanks
29. Auricle; external auditory canal, p. 236
30. Eardrum, p. 236
31. Ossicles, p. 238
32. Oval window, p. 238
33. Otitis media, p. 239
34. Vestibule, p. 239
35. Mechanoreceptors, p. 239
36. Crista ampullaris, p. 239

Circle the correct answer
37. Papillae, p. 241
38. Cranial, p. 243
39. Mucus, p. 243
40. Memory, p. 244
41. Chemoreceptors, p. 243

Unscramble the words
42. Auricle
43. Sclera
44. Papilla
45. Conjunctiva
46. Pupils

Applying what you know
47. External otitis
48. Cataracts
49. The Eustachian tube connects the throat to the middle ear and provides a perfect pathway for the spread of infection.
50. Olfactory

51.

M	E	C	H	A	N	O	R	E	C	E	P	T	O	R
H	R	A	T	B	Q	I	R	T	B	N	H	M	A	E
P	F	T	Y	R	O	T	C	A	F	L	O	X	R	C
G	U	A	Y	I	N	A	I	H	C	A	T	S	U	E
G	P	R	A	C	E	R	U	M	E	N	O	P	X	P
I	E	A	I	P	O	Y	B	S	E	R	P	K	D	T
W	L	C	P	L	Y	N	E	Y	K	E	I	T	O	O
C	Q	T	O	I	B	R	J	B	S	F	G	L	M	R
Z	U	S	R	C	L	E	O	U	J	R	M	N	N	S
F	D	M	E	O	H	L	Q	T	N	A	E	Y	I	S
H	I	D	P	N	D	L	A	M	A	C	N	X	S	Z
A	M	L	Y	E	S	S	E	E	D	T	T	M	Z	H
D	D	M	H	S	F	E	X	A	Y	I	S	I	I	A
J	C	G	N	J	T	I	S	L	P	O	G	U	V	J
P	H	G	Y	A	K	H	S	U	C	N	I	S	G	A

Crossword

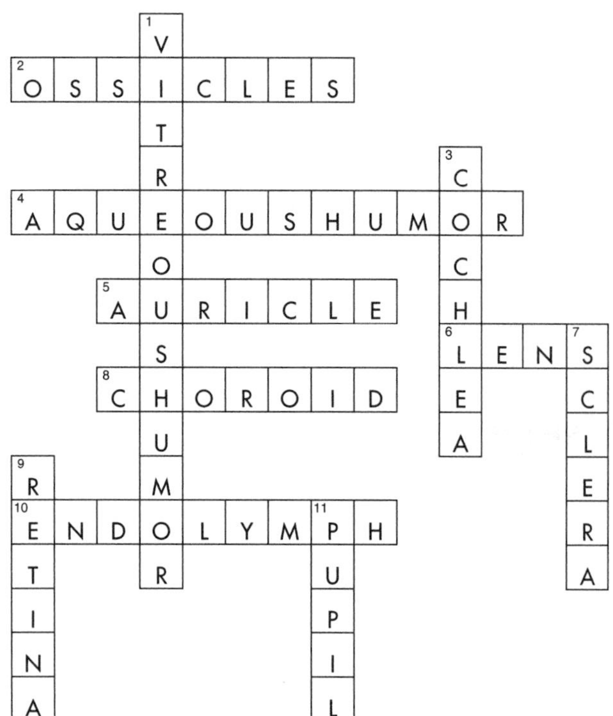

Check your knowledge

Multiple choice

1. A, p. 229
2. B, p. 236
3. A, p. 235
4. C, p. 235
5. B, p. 235
6. B, p. 239
7. D, p. 231
8. B, p. 235
9. D, p. 238
10. A, p. 234

True or false

11. T, p. 227
12. F, Window of the eye, p. 231
13. T, p. 232
14. F, Cataract, p. 234
15. T, p. 233
16. T, p. 235
17. T, p. 238
18. T, p. 239
19. T, p. 241
20. T, p. 231

Eye

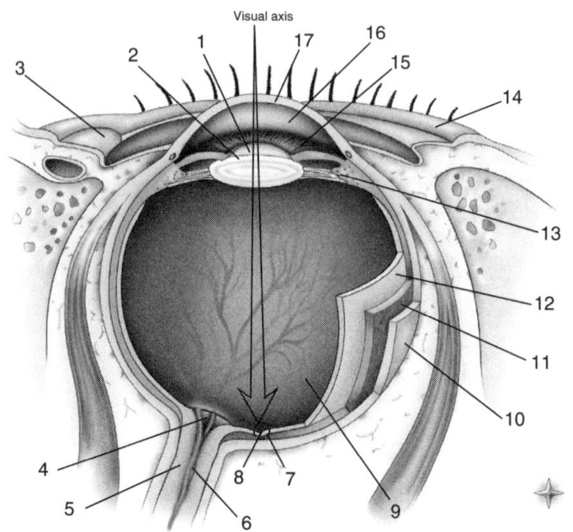

1. Pupil
2. Lens
3. Lacrimal caruncle
4. Optic disk
5. Optic nerve
6. Central artery and vein
7. Macula lutea
8. Fovea
9. Posterior chamber
10. Sclera
11. Choroid
12. Retina
13. Ciliary body
14. Lower lid
15. Iris
16. Anterior chamber
17. Cornea

Ear

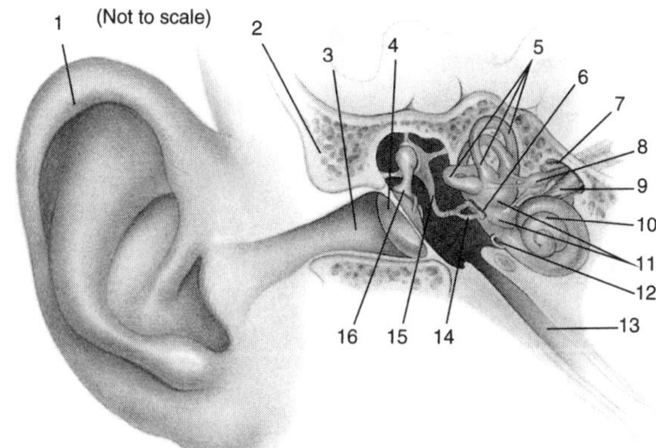

1. Auricle
2. Temporal bone
3. External auditory meatus
4. Tympanic membrane
5. Semicircular canals
6. Oval window
7. Facial nerve
8. Vestibular nerve
9. Cochlear nerve
10. Cochlea
11. Vestibule
12. Round window
13. Auditory tube
14. Stapes
15. Incus
16. Malleus

CHAPTER 10
ENDOCRINE SYSTEM

Matching

Group A
1. D, p. 251
2. C, p. 251
3. E, p. 251
4. A, p. 251
5. B, p. 251

Group B
6. E, p. 256
7. C, p. 257
8. A, p. 255
9. D, p. 251
10. B, p. 252

Fill in the blanks
11. First messengers, p. 255
12. Endocrine glands, p. 255
13. Target organs, p. 255
14. Cyclic AMP, p. 255
15. Second messenger, p. 255
16. Communication, p. 255
17. Target cells, p. 255

Circle the correct answer
18. B, p. 258
19. E, p. 258
20. D, p. 258
21. D, p. 258
22. A, p. 259
23. C, p. 259
24. C, p. 259
25. B, p. 258
26. A, p. 258
27. A, p. 258
28. D, p. 259
29. B, p. 259
30. A, p. 259
31. C, p. 260
32. C, p. 261

Select the correct term
33. A, p. 258
34. B, p. 258
35. B, p. 260
36. C, p. 261
37. A, p. 259
38. C, p. 261
39. A, p. 258
40. A, p. 258
41. A, p. 259
42. C, p. 261

Circle the correct answer
43. Below, p. 261
44. Calcitonin, p. 261
45. Iodine, p. 261
46. Do not, p. 261
47. Thyroid, p. 261
48. Decrease, p. 261
49. Hypothyroidism, p. 264
50. Cretinism, p. 264
51. PTH, p. 261
52. Increase, p. 262

Fill in the blanks
53. Adrenal cortex; adrenal medulla, p. 263
54. Corticoids, p. 263
55. Mineralocorticoids, p. 263
56. Glucocorticoids, p. 264
57. Sex hormones, p. 264
58. Gluconeogenesis, p. 265
59. Blood pressure, p. 265
60. Epinephrine; norepinephrine, p. 266
61. Stress, p. 266
62. Addison's disease, p. 267

Select the correct term
63. A, p. 264
64. A, p. 265
65. B, p. 266
66. A, p. 267
67. B, p. 266
68. A, p. 264
69. A, p. 266

Circle the term that does not belong
70. Beta cells (all others refer to glucagon)
71. Glucagon (all others refer to insulin)
72. Thymosin (all others refer to female sex glands)
73. Chorion (all other refer to male sex glands)
74. Aldosterone (all others refer to the thymus)
75. ACTH (all others refer to the placenta)
76. Semen (all others refer to the pineal gland)

Matching

Group A
77. E, p. 268
78. C, p. 268
79. B, p. 271
80. D, p. 271
81. A, p. 271

Group B
82. E, p. 271
83. A, p. 271
84. B, p. 272
85. C, p. 271
86. D, p. 271

Unscramble the words

87. Corticoids
88. Diuresis
89. Glucocorticoids
90. Steroids
91. Stress

Applying what you know

92. She was pregnant.
93. Adrenal cortex (This source of testosterone may produce secondary male characteristics if unattended to at this young age.)
94. Oxytocin

95.

S	S	I	S	E	R	U	I	D	M	E	S	I	T	W
N	D	N	X	E	B	A	M	E	D	E	X	Y	M	I
I	I	G	O	N	R	S	G	X	T	I	I	Y	V	B
D	O	M	S	I	N	I	T	E	R	C	C	U	Q	D
N	C	X	S	R	T	N	B	O	T	V	M	Y	O	M
A	I	M	E	C	L	A	C	R	E	P	Y	H	I	X
L	T	Y	R	O	I	E	Z	Q	R	T	J	V	K	F
G	R	E	T	D	P	S	N	I	L	D	J	M	X	N
A	O	O	S	N	I	D	K	I	N	K	S	P	P	O
T	C	P	R	E	T	I	O	G	R	I	F	M	X	G
S	L	M	H	Y	P	O	G	L	Y	C	E	M	I	A
O	A	J	L	H	O	R	M	O	N	E	O	T	G	C
R	C	E	L	T	S	E	L	C	N	P	N	X	U	U
P	I	O	S	W	R	T	X	C	G	U	L	O	E	L
G	G	V	Y	H	M	S	H	Y	K	A	K	N	Q	G

Crossword

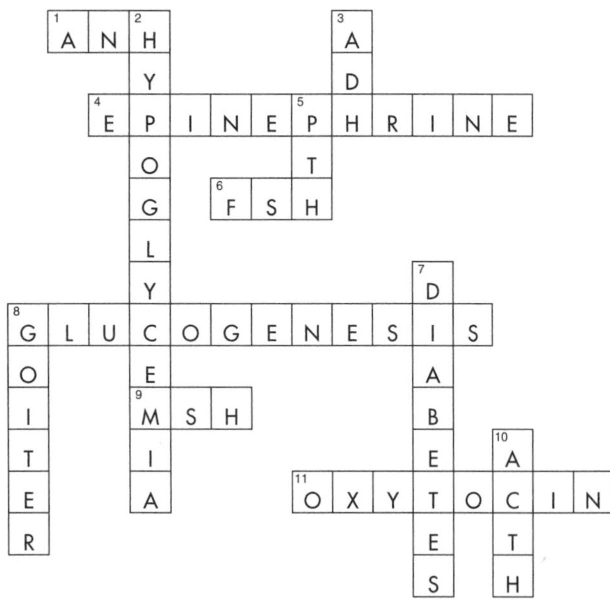

Check your knowledge

Multiple choice

1. A, p. 251
2. C, p. 258
3. D, p. 257
4. C, p. 259
5. D, p. 259
6. D, p. 260
7. B, p. 261
8. D, p. 266
9. D, p. 271
10. B, p. 271

Matching

11. J, p. 255
12. G, p. 257
13. H, p. 258
14. I, p. 264
15. B, p. 264
16. F, p. 264
17. A, p. 268
18. D, p. 269
19. E, p. 271
20. C, p. 258

Endocrine glands

1. Pineal
2. Hypothalamus
3. Pituitary
4. Thyroid
5. Thymus
6. Adrenals
7. Pancreas (islets)
8. Ovaries (female)
9. Testes (male)
10. Parathyroids

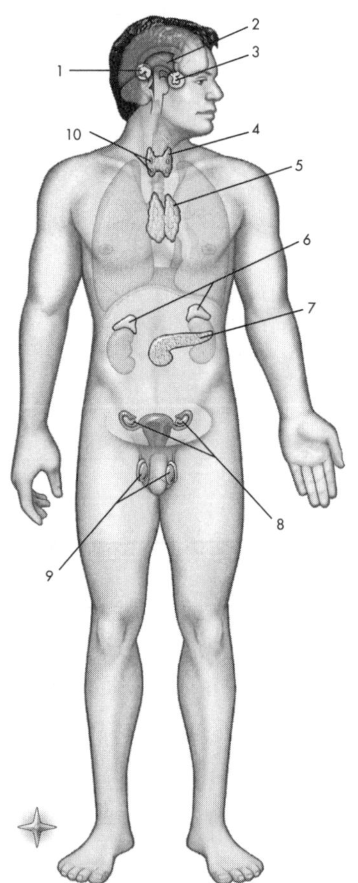

CHAPTER 11
BLOOD

Circle the correct answer

1. E, p. 282
2. D, p. 283
3. D, p. 283
4. B, p. 283
5. C, p. 283
6. A, p. 285
7. B, p. 286
8. D, p. 283
9. C, p. 283
10. D, p. 286
11. A, p. 285
12. B, p. 293
13. B, p. 291
14. B, p. 283
15. E, p. 284
16. B, p. 284
17. C, p. 284
18. D, p. 284
19. D, p. 286
20. D, p. 286
21. B, p. 288
22. D, p. 284
23. B, p. 288
24. C, p. 288
25. B, p. 288
26. A, p. 291
27. E, p. 291

Fill in the missing areas

28.

Blood Type	Antigen	Antibody
A	A	
B		Anti-A
AB	A, B	
O		Anti-A, Anti-B

Fill in the blanks

29. Antigen, p. 291
30. Antibody, p. 291
31. Agglutinate, p. 291
32. Erythroblastosis fetalis, p. 294
33. Rhesus monkey, p. 293
34. RhoGAM, p. 294
35. AB positive, p. 293

Applying what you know

36. No. If Mrs. Lassiter had a negative Rh factor and her husband had a positive Rh factor, it would set up the strong possibility of erythroblastosis fetalis.
37. Both procedures assist the clotting process.

38.

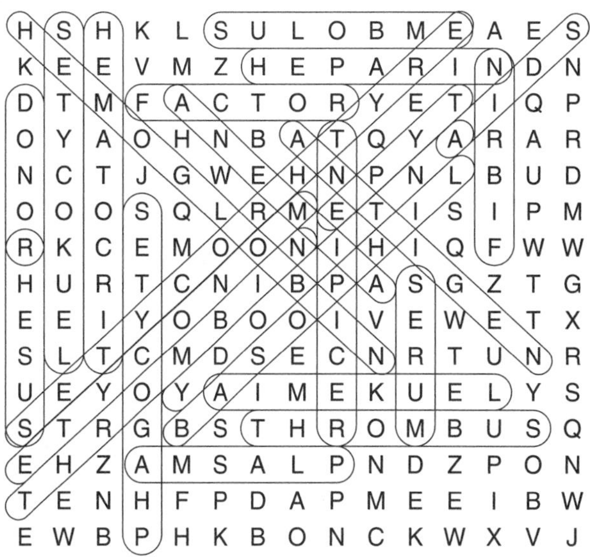

Crossword

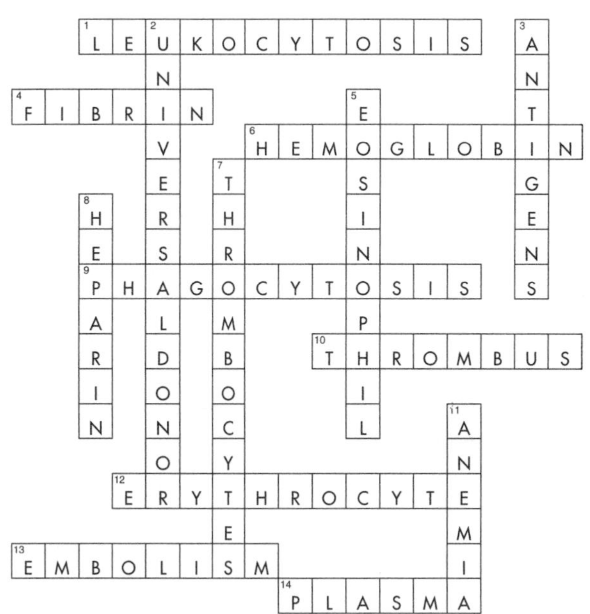

Check your knowledge

Multiple choice

1. B, p. 281
2. B, p. 282
3. A, p. 283
4. A, p. 286
5. D, p. 289
6. A, p. 287
7. A, p. 291
8. D, p. 291

9. C, p. 293
10. B, p. 294

Matching
11. D, p. 282
12. F, p. 284
13. H, p. 284
14. A, p. 286
15. G, p. 287
16. C, p. 288
17. B, p. 288
18. E, p. 286
19. I, p. 288
20. J, p. 291

Human blood cells

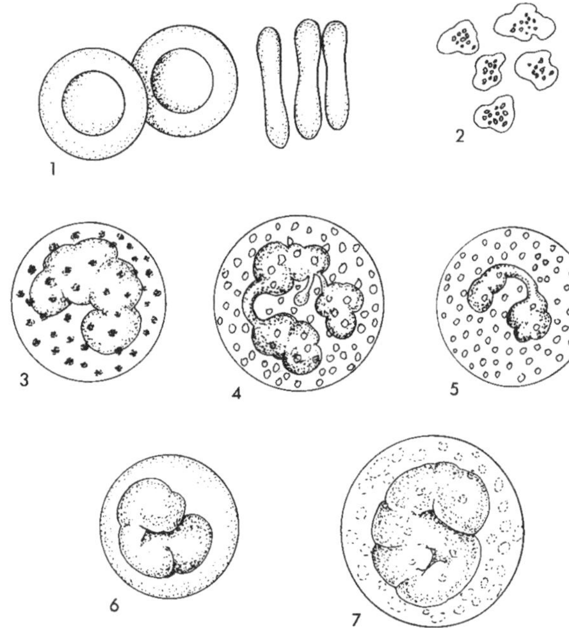

1. Red blood cells
2. Platelets
3. Basophil
4. Neutrophil
5. Eosinophil
6. Lymphocyte
7. Monocyte

Blood typing

Recipient's blood		*Reactions with donor's blood*			
RBC antigens	Plasma antibodies	Donor type O	Donor type A	Donor type B	Donor type AB
None (Type O)	Anti-A Anti-B	Normal blood	Agglutinated blood	Agglutinated blood	Agglutinated blood
A (Type A)	Anti-B	Normal blood	Normal blood	Agglutinated blood	Agglutinated blood
B (Type B)	Anti-A	Normal blood	Agglutinated blood	Normal blood	Agglutinated blood
AB (Type AB)	(none)	Normal blood	Normal blood	Normal blood	Normal blood

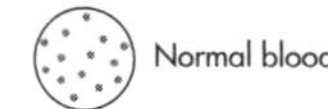 Normal blood 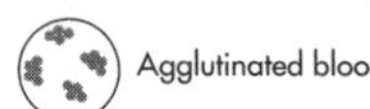 Agglutinated blood

CHAPTER 12 THE CIRCULATORY SYSTEM

Fill in the blanks
1. CPR, p. 302
2. Interatrial septum, p. 302
3. Atria, p. 302
4. Ventricles, p. 302
5. Myocardium, p. 302
6. Endocarditis, p. 302
7. Bicuspid or mitral; tricuspid, p. 305
8. Pulmonary circulation, p. 307
9. Coronary embolism or coronary thrombosis, p. 307
10. Myocardial infarction, p. 307
11. Sinoatrial, p. 310
12. P; QRS complex; T, p. 310
13. Repolarization, p. 310

Choose the correct term
14. A, p. 305
15. K, p. 302
16. G, p. 307
17. C, p. 307
18. D, p. 305
19. F, p. 302
20. H, p. 307
21. B, p. 307
22. E, p. 310
23. I, p. 305
24. J, p. 310
25. L, p. 302
26. M, p. 305

Matching
27. D, p. 315
28. B, p. 315
29. C, p. 315

30. G, p. 313
31. A, p. 315
32. E, p. 313
33. F, p. 311

Multiple choice

34. D, p. 315
35. C, p. 315
36. B, p. 314
37. A, p. 131
38. B, p. 311
39. B, p. 315
40. D, p. 317
41. B, p. 319
42. B, p. 319
43. A, p. 319
44. D, p. 313
45. A, p. 314

True or false

46. Highest in arteries, lowest in veins, p. 320
47. Blood pressure gradient, p. 320
48. Stop, p. 320
49. High, p. 320
50. Decreases, p. 320
51. T
52. T
53. T
54. Stronger will increase, weaker will decrease, p. 322
55. Contract, p. 326
56. Relax, p. 326
57. Artery, p. 326
58. T
59. T
60. Brachial, p. 327

Unscramble the words

61. Systemic
62. Venule
63. Artery
64. Pulse
65. Vessel

Applying what you know

66. Coronary bypass surgery
67. Artificial pacemaker
68. The endocardial lining can become rough and abrasive to red blood cells passing over its surface. As a result, a fatal blood clot may be formed.
69. Dan may be hemorrhaging. The heart beats faster during hemorrhage in an attempt to compensate for blood loss.

70.

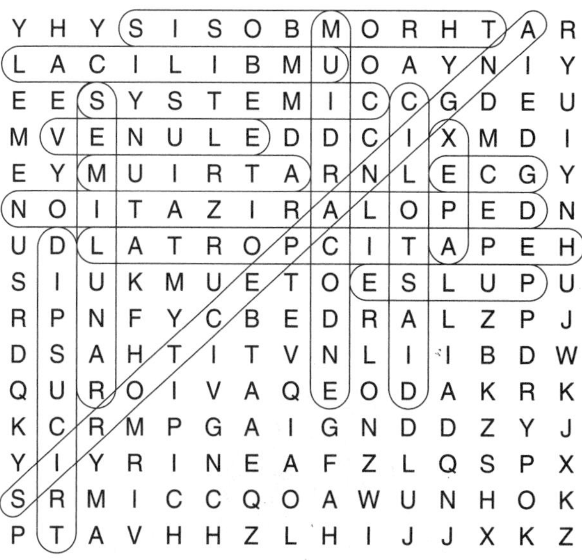

Crossword

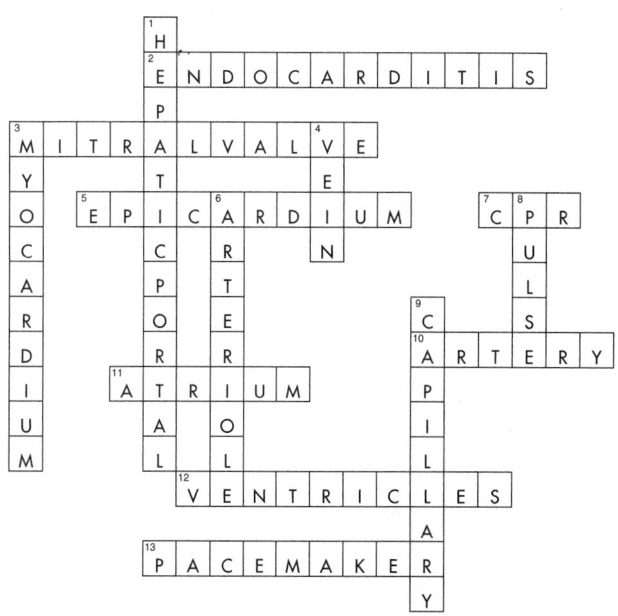

Check your knowledge

Multiple choice

1. A, p. 302
2. C, p. 305
3. B, p. 315
4. A, p. 310
5. A, p. 313
6. D, p. 310
7. C, p. 320
8. D, p. 319
9. C, p. 308
10. C, p. 314

Matching

11. F, p. 302
12. G, p. 305
13. H, p. 305
14. I, p. 307
15. J, p. 311
16. B, p. 310
17. C, p. 302
18. A, p. 326
19. D, p. 328
20. E, p. 326

The heart

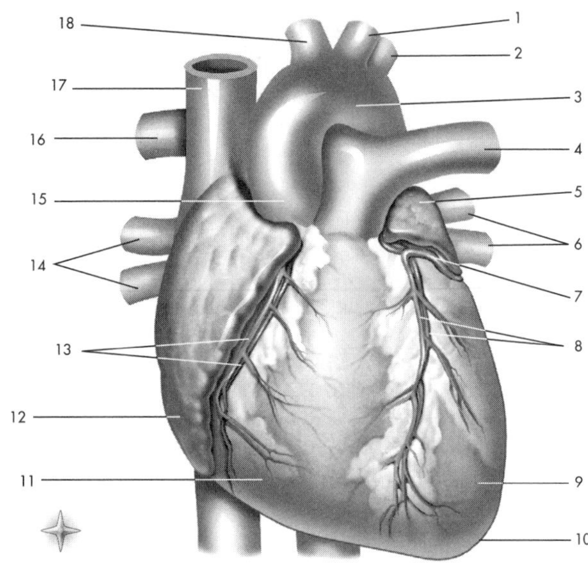

1. Left common carotid artery
2. Left subclavian artery
3. Arch of aorta
4. Left pulmonary artery
5. Left atrium
6. Left pulmonary veins
7. Great cardiac vein
8. Branches of left coronary artery and cardiac vein
9. Left ventricle
10. Apex
11. Right ventricle
12. Right atrium
13. Right coronary artery and cardiac vein
14. Right pulmonary veins
15. Ascending aorta
16. Right pulmonary artery
17. Superior vena cava
18. Brachiocephalic trunk

Conduction system of the heart

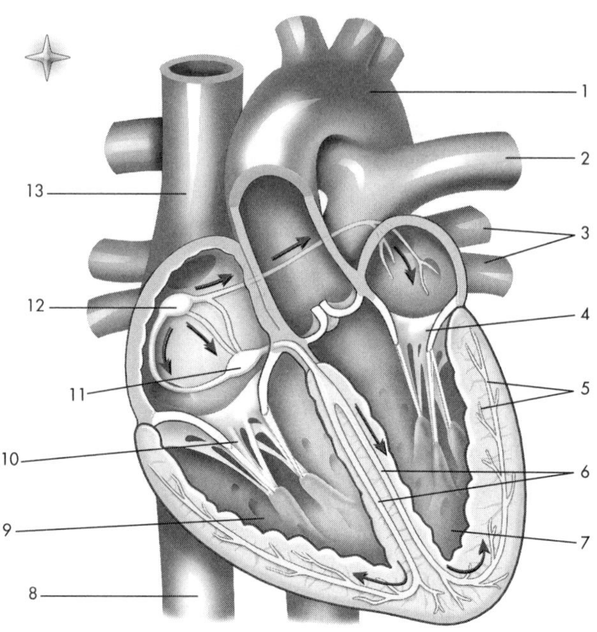

1. Aorta
2. Pulmonary artery
3. Pulmonary veins
4. Mitral (bicuspid) valve
5. Purkinje fibers
6. Right and left branches of AV bundle (bundle of His)
7. Left ventricle
8. Inferior vena cava
9. Right ventricle
10. Tricuspid valve
11. Atrioventricular (AV) node
12. Sinoatrial (SA) node or pacemaker
13. Superior vena cava

Fetal circulation

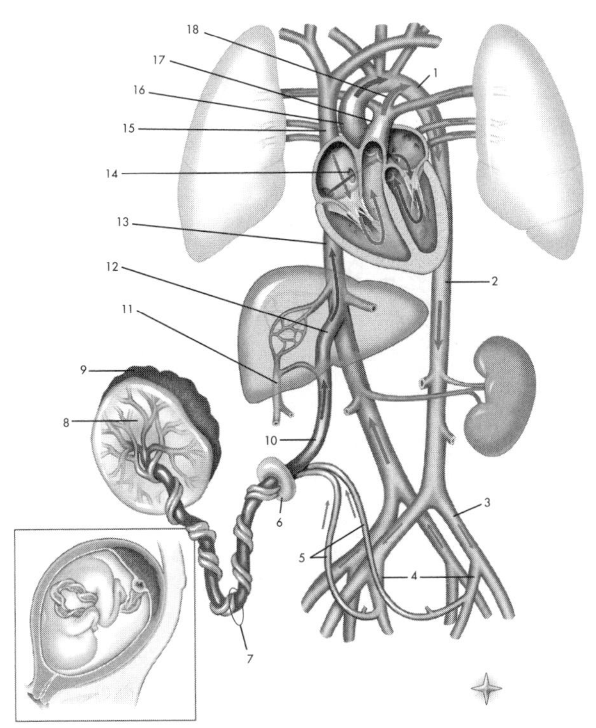

1. Aortic arch
2. Abdominal aorta
3. Common iliac artery
4. Internal iliac arteries
5. Umbilical arteries
6. Fetal umbilicus
7. Umbilical cord
8. Fetal side of placenta
9. Maternal side of placenta
10. Umbilical vein
11. Hepatic portal vein
12. Ductus venosus
13. Inferior vena cava
14. Foramen ovale
15. Superior vena cava
16. Ascending aorta
17. Pulmonary trunk
18. Ductus arteriosus

Hepatic portal circulation

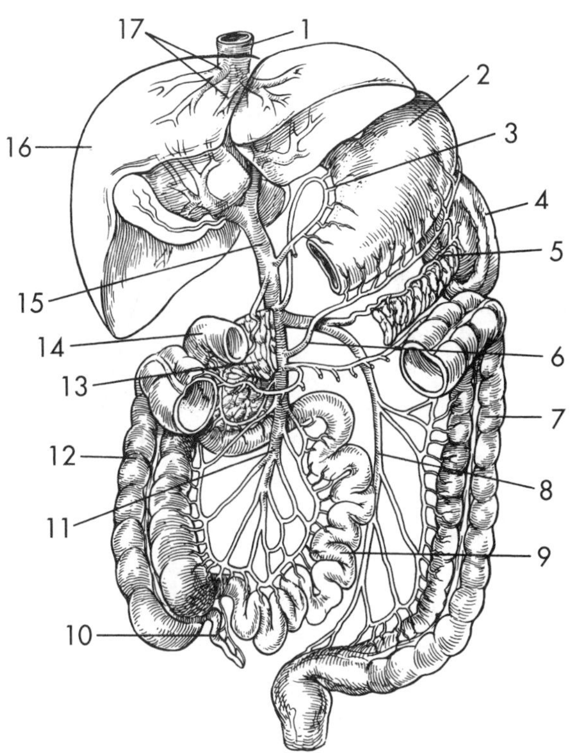

1. Inferior vena cava
2. Stomach
3. Gastric vein
4. Spleen
5. Splenic vein
6. Gastroepiploic vein
7. Descending colon
8. Inferior mesenteric vein
9. Small intestine
10. Appendix
11. Superior mesenteric vein
12. Ascending colon
13. Pancreas
14. Duodenum
15. Hepatic portal vein
16. Liver
17. Hepatic veins

Principal arteries of the body

1. Right common carotid
2. Brachiocephalic
3. Right coronary
4. Axillary
5. Brachial
6. Superior mesenteric
7. Abdominal aorta
8. Common iliac
9. Internal iliac
10. External iliac
11. Deep femoral
12. Femoral
13. Popliteal
14. Anterior tibia
15. Occipital
16. Facial
17. Internal carotid
18. External carotid
19. Left common carotid
20. Left subclavian
21. Arch of aorta
22. Pulmonary
23. Left coronary
24. Aorta
25. Splenic
26. Renal
27. Celiac
28. Inferior mesenteric
29. Radial
30. Ulnar

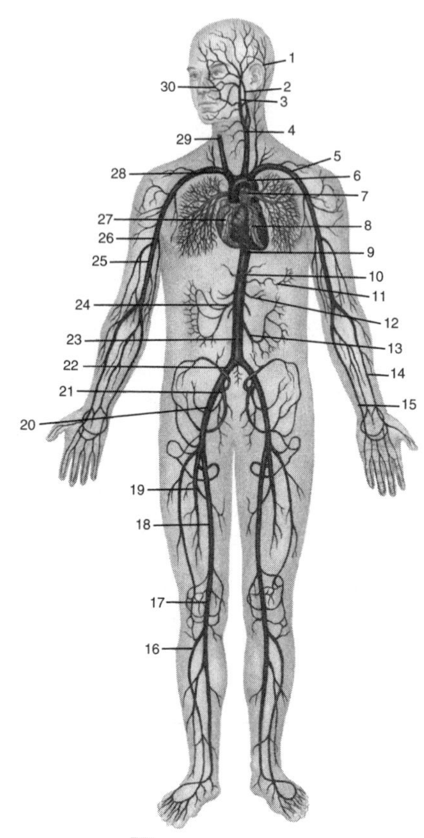

Principal veins of the body

1. Right brachiocephalic
2. Right subclavian
3. Superior vena cava
4. Right pulmonary
5. Small cardiac
6. Inferior vena cava
7. Hepatic
8. Hepatic portal
9. Superior mesenteric
10. Median cubital
11. Common iliac
12. External iliac
13. Femoral
14. Great saphenous
15. Fibular
16. Anterior tibial
17. Posterior tibial
18. Occipital
19. Facial
20. External jugular
21. Internal jugular
22. Left brachiocephalic
23. Left subclavian
24. Axillary
25. Cephalic
26. Great cardiac
27. Basilic
28. Long thoracic
29. Splenic
30. Inferior mesenteric
31. Common iliac
32. Internal iliac
33. Femoral
34. Popliteal

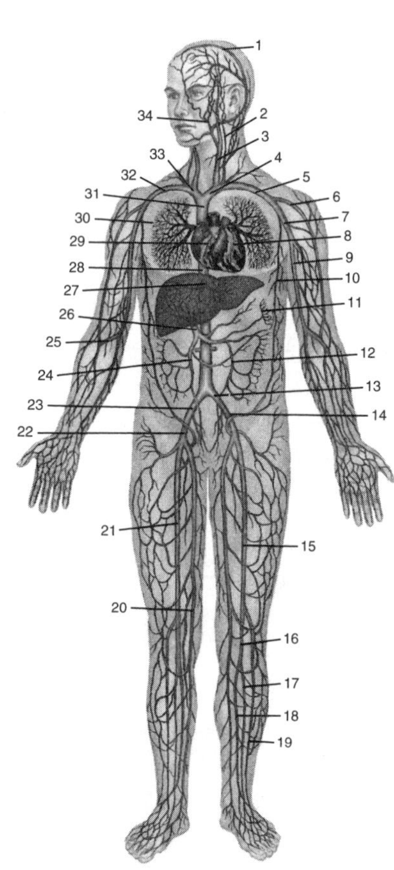

Normal ECG deflections

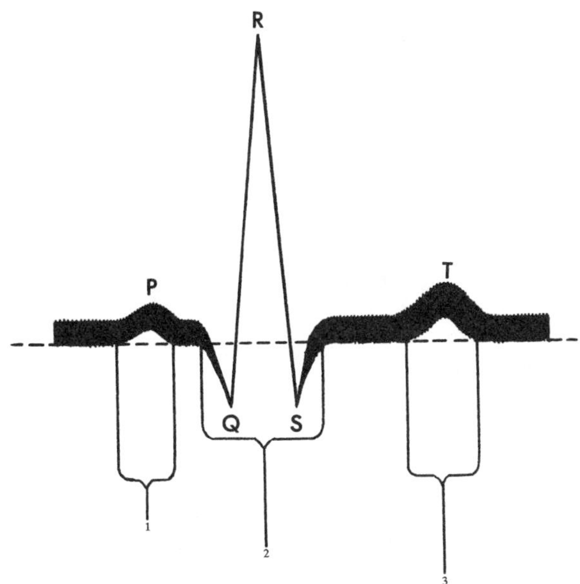

1. Atrial depolarization
2. Ventricular depolarization
3. Ventricular repolarization

CHAPTER 13
THE LYMPHATIC SYSTEM AND IMMUNITY

Fill in the blanks

1. Lymph, p. 338
2. Interstitial fluid, p. 338
3. Lymphatic capillaries, p. 338
4. Right lymphatic duct; thoracic duct, p. 339
5. Cisterna chyli, p. 339
6. Lymph nodes, p. 339
7. Afferent, p. 339
8. Efferent, p. 340

Select the correct term

9. B, p. 342
10. C, p. 342
11. C, p. 343
12. A, p. 341
13. C, p. 343
14. A, p. 342
15. A, p. 341

Matching

16. C, p. 344
17. A, p. 345
18. E, p. 345
19. B, p. 345
20. D, p. 345

Choose the correct term

21. C, p. 343
22. D, p. 343
23. E, p. 348
24. A, p. 346
25. H, p. 346
26. B, p. 346
27. I, p. 346
28. F, p. 347
29. J, p. 348
30. G, p. 347

Circle the one that does not belong

31. Allergy (all others refer to antibodies)
32. Complement (all others refer to antigens)
33. Antigen (all others refer to monoclonal antibodies)
34. Complement (all others refer to allergy)
35. Monoclonal (all others refer to complement)

Multiple choice

36. D, p. 349
37. D, p. 351
38. C, p. 351
39. B, p. 340
40. C, p. 352
41. C, p. 349
42. E, p. 350
43. E, p. 352
44. C, p. 352
45. E, p. 352
46. E, p. 353
47. D, p. 352
48. E, p. 349
49. A, p. 352
50. B, p. 353

Fill in the blanks

51. Stem cell, p. 349
52. Activated B cell, p. 350
53. Plasma cells, p. 352
54. Thymus gland, p. 353
55. Azidothymidine or AZT, p. 352
56. AIDS, p. 352
57. Vaccine, p. 352

Unscramble the words

58. Complement
59. Immunity
60. Clones
61. Interferon
62. Memory cells

Applying what you know

63. Interferon would possibly decrease the severity of the chickenpox virus.

64. AIDS
65. Baby Phelps had no means of producing T cells, thus making him susceptible to several diseases. Isolation was a means of controlling his exposure to these diseases.

66.

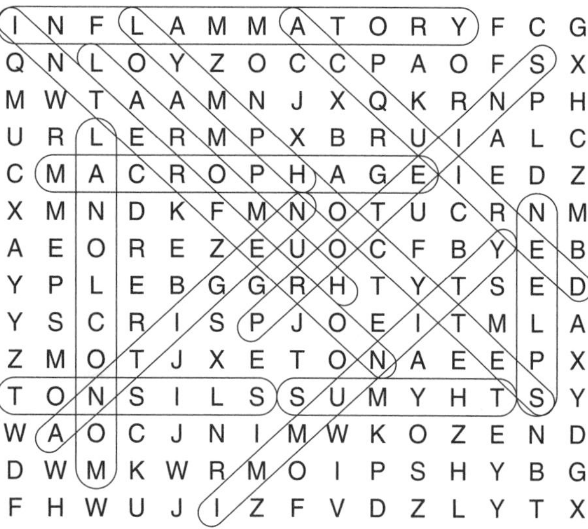

Crossword

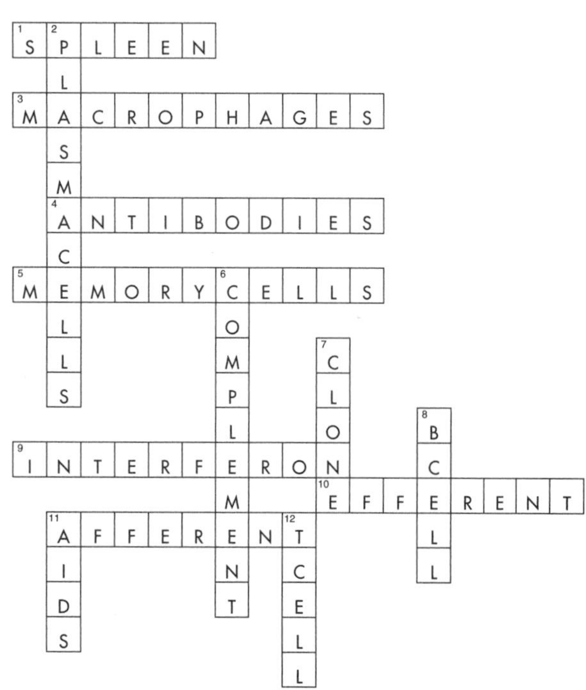

Check your knowledge

Multiple choice

1. A, p. 338
2. A, p. 342
3. D, p. 339
4. B, p. 340
5. D, p. 341
6. B, p. 342
7. D, p. 345
8. D, p. 353
9. D, p. 344
10. C, p. 346

Matching

11. E, p. 340
12. D, p. 342
13. I, p. 344
14. H, p. 345
15. G, p. 346
16. B, p. 343
17. A, p. 346
18. J, p. 348
19. C, p. 349
20. F, p. 349

Principal organs of the lymphatic system

1. Cervical lymph nodes
2. Submandibular nodes
3. Thymus
4. Axillary lymph nodes
5. Thoracic duct
6. Spleen
7. Cisterna chyli
8. Inguinal lymph nodes
9. Popliteal lymph nodes
10. Lymph vessels
11. Red bone marrow
12. Right lymphatic duct

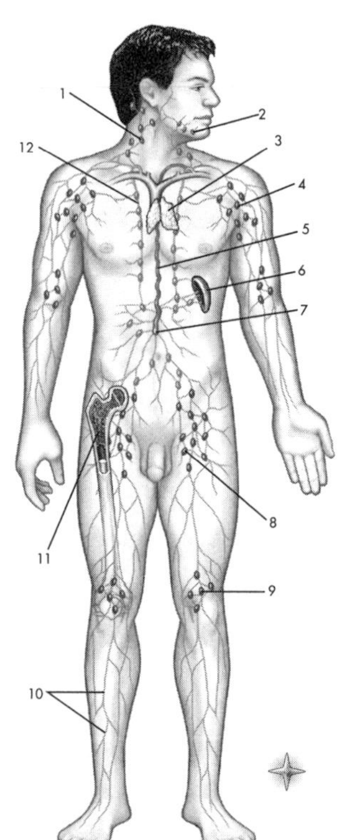

CHAPTER 14 THE RESPIRATORY SYSTEM

Matching

1. J, p. 361
2. G, p. 364
3. A, p. 362
4. I, p. 365
5. B, p. 364
6. F, p. 364

7. C, p. 362
8. H, p. 364
9. D, p. 364
10. E, p. 361

Fill in the blanks

11. Air distributor, p. 361
12. Gas exchanger, p. 361
13. Filters, p. 361
14. Warms, p. 361
15. Humidifies, p. 361
16. Nose, p. 362
17. Pharynx, p. 362
18. Larynx, p. 362
19. Trachea, p. 362
20. Bronchi, p. 362
21. Lungs, p. 362
22. Alveoli, p. 362
23. Diffusion, p. 362
24. Respiratory membrane, p. 364
25. Respiratory mucosa, p. 364

Circle the one that does not belong

26. Oropharynx (the others refer to the nose)
27. Conchae (the others refer to paranasal sinuses)
28. Epiglottis (the others refer to the pharynx)
29. Uvula (the others refer to the adenoids)
30. Larynx (the others refer to the eustachian tubes)
31. Tonsils (the others refer to the larynx)
32. Eustachian tube (the others refer to the tonsils)
33. Pharynx (the others refer to the larynx)

Choose the correct term

34. A, p. 365
35. B, p. 366
36. A, p. 365
37. A, p. 365
38. A, p. 365
39. B, p. 366
40. B, p. 366
41. C, p. 368

Fill in the blanks

42. Trachea, p. 368
43. Cartilage (C-rings), p. 369
44. Suffocation, p. 370
45. Primary bronchi, p. 370
46. Alveolar sacs, p. 370
47. Apex, p. 371
48. Pleura, p. 373
49. Pleurisy, p. 373
50. Pneumothorax, p. 373

True or false

51. Breathing, p. 374
52. Expiration, p. 376
53. Down, p. 377 (review Chapter 3)
54. Internal, p. 377
55. T
56. 1 pint, p. 380
57. T
58. Vital capacity, p. 380
59. T

Circle the correct answer

60. E, p. 374
61. C, p. 379
62. C, p. 379
63. B, p. 376
64. D, p. 380
65. D, p. 380
66. D, p. 380

Matching

67. E, p. 382
68. B, p. 382
69. G, p. 383
70. A, p. 384
71. F, p. 384
72. D, p. 384
73. C, p. 384

Unscramble the words

74. Pleurisy
75. Bronchitis
76. Epistaxis
77. Adenoids
78. Inspiration

Applying what you know

79. During the day Mr. Gorski's cilia are paralyzed because of his heavy smoking. They use the time when Mr. Gorski is asleep to sweep accumulations of mucus and bacteria toward the pharynx. When he awakes, these collections are waiting to be eliminated.
80. Swelling of the tonsils or adenoids caused by infection may make it difficult or impossible for air to travel from the nose into the throat. The individual may be forced to breathe through the mouth.

81.

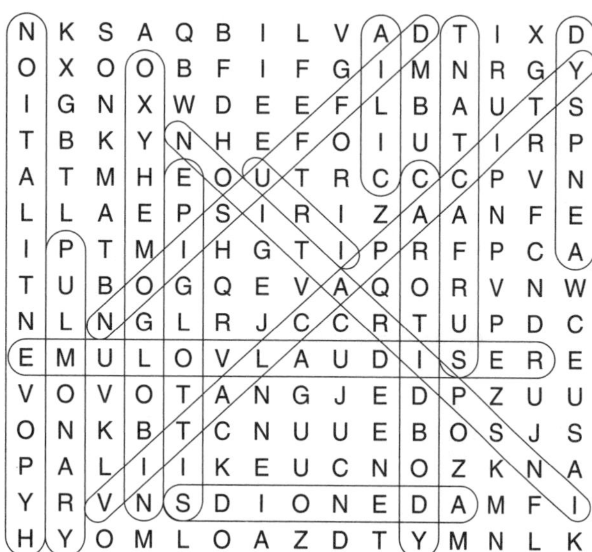

Crossword

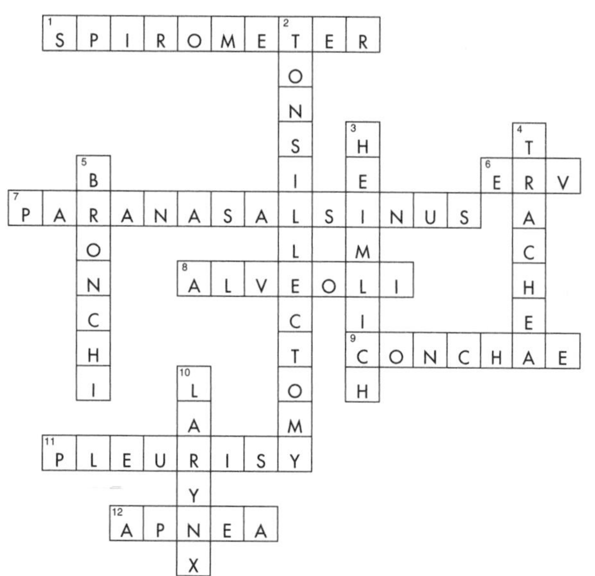

Check your knowledge

Multiple choice

1. A, p. 362
2. B, p. 365
3. D, p. 361
4. B, p. 370
5. A, p. 376
6. D, p. 373
7. A, p. 377
8. C, p. 380
9. D, p. 384
10. B, p. 382

Matching

11. E, p. 364
12. I, p. 364
13. A, p. 365
14. G, p. 368
15. D, p. 369
16. B, p. 380
17. C, p. 382
18. H, p. 384
19. F, p. 384
20. J, p. 371

Sagittal view of head and neck

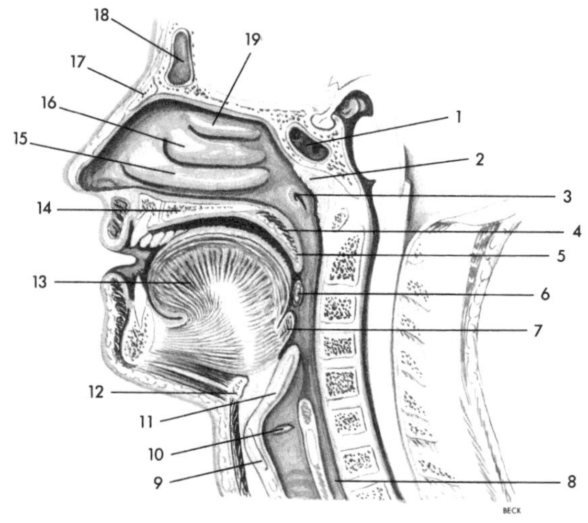

1. Sphenoidal air sinus
2. Pharyngeal tonsil (adenoids)
3. Auditory tube
4. Soft palate
5. Uvula
6. Palatine tonsil
7. Lingual tonsil
8. Esophagus
9. Thyroid cartilage
10. Vocal cords
11. Epiglottis
12. Hyoid bone
13. Tongue
14. Hard palate
15. Inferior concha
16. Middle concha
17. Nasal bone
18. Frontal air sinus
19. Superior concha

Respiratory organs

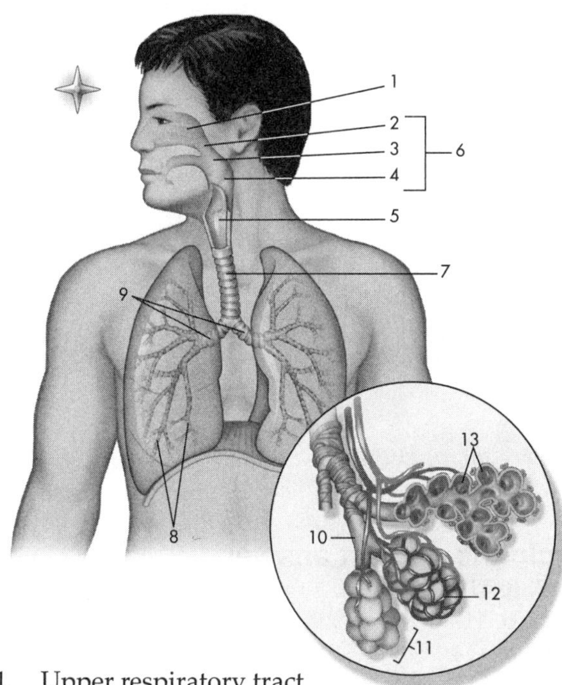

1. Upper respiratory tract
2. Lower respiratory tract
3. Left and right primary bronchi
4. Bronchioles
5. Nasal cavity
6. Nasopharynx
7. Oropharynx
8. Laryngopharynx
9. Larynx
10. Pharynx
11. Trachea
12. Alveolar duct
13. Alveolar sac
14. Capillary
15. Alveoli

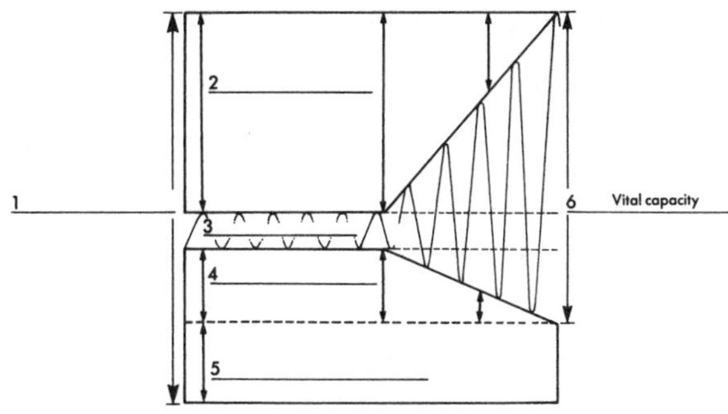

Pulmonary ventilation volumes

1. Total lung capacity
2. Inspiratory reserve volume
3. Tidal volume
4. Expiratory reserve volume
5. Residual volume

CHAPTER 15 THE DIGESTIVE SYSTEM

Fill in the blanks

1. Gastrointestinal tract or GI tract, p. 391
2. Mechanical, p. 391
3. Chemical, p. 391
4. Feces, p. 392
5. Digestion; absorption; metabolism, p. 392
6. Visceral peritoneum, p. 392
7. Mouth; anus, p. 392
8. Lumen, p. 392
9. Mucosa, p. 392
10. Submucosa, p. 392
11. Peristalsis, p. 392
12. Serosa, p. 392
13. Mesentery, p. 392

Choose the correct term

14. A, p. 392
15. B, p. 392
16. B, p. 392
17. A, p. 392
18. A, p. 392
19. A, p. 392
20. A, p. 392
21. A, p. 392
22. B, p. 392
23. B, p. 392
24. B, p. 392
25. B, p. 392

Circle the correct answer

26. E, p. 393
27. C, p. 394
28. E, p. 396
29. D, p. 395
30. B, p. 395
31. C, p. 398
32. D, p. 398
33. D, p. 397
34. D, p. 395
35. A, p. 397
36. C, p. 397
37. A, p. 397
38. A, p. 395
39. B, p. 398
40. C, p. 396

Fill in the blanks

41. Pharynx, p. 398
42. Esophagus, p. 398
43. Stomach, p. 398
44. Cardiac sphincter, p. 399
45. Chyme, p. 399

46. Fundus, p. 400
47. Body, p. 400
48. Pylorus, p. 400
49. Pyloric sphincter, p. 400
50. Small intestine, p. 400

Matching

51. D, p. 400
52. J, p. 400
53. G, p. 399
54. A, p. 399
55. H, p. 401
56. B, p. 399
57. C, p. 400
58. E, p. 403
59. I, p. 401
60. F, p. 400

Circle the correct answer

61. C, p. 403
62. B, p. 400 and p. 403
63. A, p. 406
64. A, p. 406
65. B, p. 403
66. E, p. 404
67. D, p. 403
68. D, p. 404; review Chapter 10 (hormones circulate in blood)
69. B, p. 406
70. C, p. 404

True or false

71. Vitamin K, p. 407
72. No villi are present in the large intestine, p. 407
73. Diarrhea, p. 407
74. Cecum, p. 408
75. Hepatic, p. 408
76. Sigmoid, p. 410
77. T
78. T
79. Parietal, p. 410
80. Mesentery, p. 410

Circle the correct answer

81. B, p. 414
82. D, p. 413
83. C, p. 414
84. C, p. 413
85. C, p. 413

86. Fill in the blank areas on the chart below.

DIGESTIVE JUICES AND ENZYMES	SUBSTANCE DIGESTED (OR HYDROLYZED)	RESULTING PRODUCT
Saliva		
	1. Starch (polysaccharide)	
Gastric juice		
		2. Partially digested proteins
Pancreatic juice		
		3. Peptides and amino acids
	4. Fats emulsified by bile	
	5. Starch	
Intestinal enzymes		
	6. Peptides	
	7. Sucrase	
	8. Lactose (milk sugar)	
		9. Glucose

Unscramble the words

87. Bolus
88. Chyme
89. Papilla
90. Peritoneum
91. Lace apron

Applying what you know

92. Ulcer
93. Pylorospasm
94. Basal metabolic rate or protein-bound iodine to determine thyroid function

95.

```
X M E T A B O L I S M X X W
R S D P E R I S T A L S I S
E V A M N O I T S E G I D R
E D E E U O Q T W Q O H N Q
Q Z H S R N I N T F E C E S
D H R E C C I T K C J A P E
Q W R N A T N V P Y R M P C
O C A T N R B A P R H O A I
U Y I E O W T A P A O T W D
B O D R L N P B F Q J S V N
N T S Y F I S L U M E E B U
W G J A L U V U N R N W O A
Q S N L X D U O D E N U M J
H C A V I T Y M U C O S A D
Y E A A P H V W S V C Q J C
```

Crossword

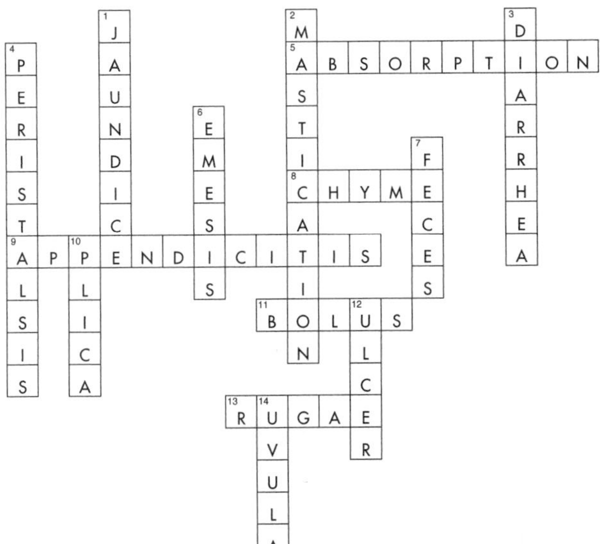

Check your knowledge

Multiple choice

1. A, p. 391
2. C, p. 392
3. A, p. 392
4. B, p. 395
5. B, p. 397
6. B, p. 396
7. B, p. 400
8. C, p. 399
9. C, p. 404
10. A, p. 406

Completion

11. Ileocecal valve, p. 406
12. Sigmoid colon, p. 407
13. Cecum, p. 410
14. Mesentery, p. 410
15. Mechanical digestion, p. 412
16. Monosaccharides, p. 413
17. Amino acids, p. 413
18. Fatty acids, glycerol, p. 413
19. Absorption, p. 413
20. Maltase, sucrase, lactase, p. 413

Digestive organs

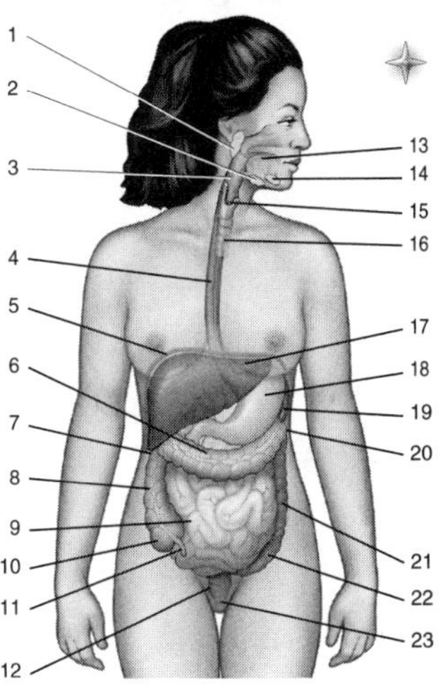

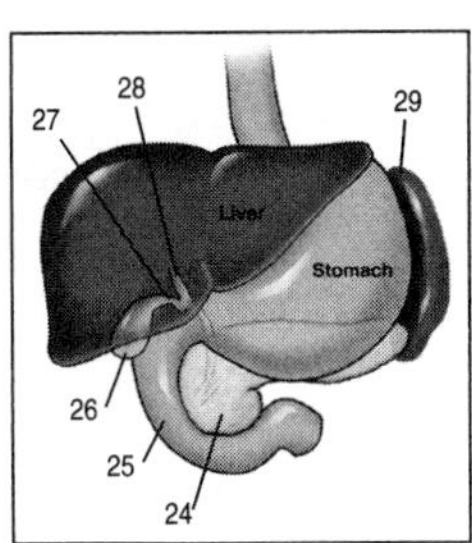

1. Parotid gland
2. Submandibular gland
3. Pharynx
4. Esophagus
5. Diaphragm
6. Transverse colon
7. Hepatic flexure
8. Ascending colon
9. Ilium
10. Cecum
11. Vermiform appendix
12. Rectum
13. Tongue
14. Sublingual gland
15. Larynx
16. Trachea
17. Liver
18. Stomach
19. Spleen
20. Splenic flexure
21. Descending colon
22. Sigmoid colon
23. Anal canal

Tooth

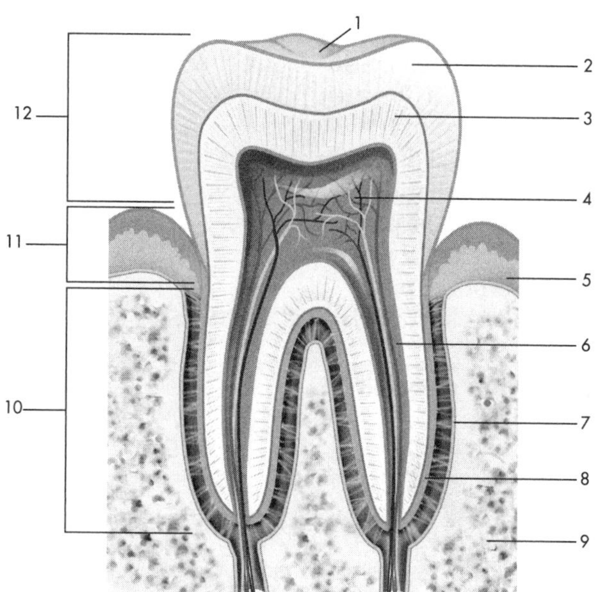

1. Cusp
2. Enamel
3. Dentin
4. Pulp cavity with nerves and vessels
5. Gingiva
6. Root canal
7. Peridontal membrane
8. Cementum
9. Bone
10. Root
11. Neck
12. Crown

The salivary glands

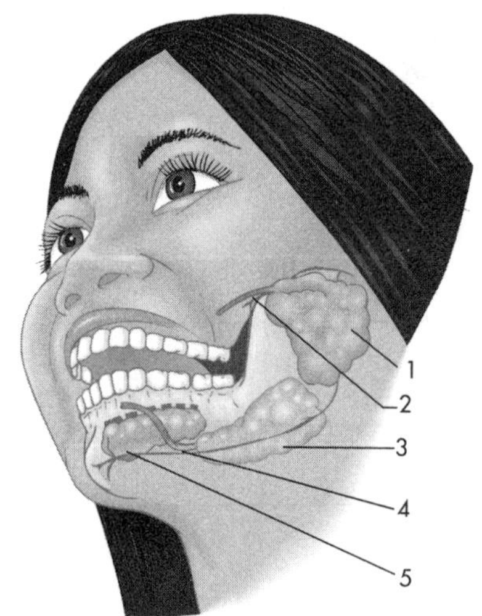

1. Parotid gland
2. Parotid duct
3. Submandibular gland
4. Submandibular duct
5. Sublingual gland

Stomach

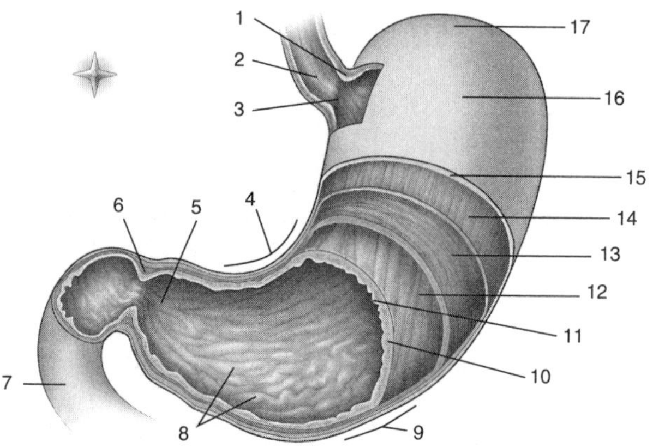

1. Gastroesophageal sphincter
2. Esophagus
3. Gastroesophageal opening
4. Lesser curvature
5. Pylorus
6. Pyloric sphincter
7. Duodenum
8. Rugae
9. Greater curvature
10. Submucosa
11. Mucosa
12. Oblique muscle layer
13. Circular muscle layer
14. Longitudinal muscle layer
15. Serosa
16. Body
17. Fundus

Gall bladder and bile ducts

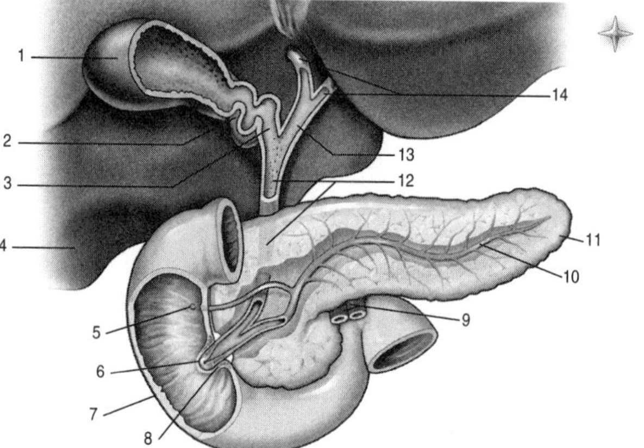

1. Corpus (body) of gallbladder
2. Neck of gallbladder
3. Cystic duct
4. Liver
5. Minor duodenal papilla
6. Major duodenal papilla
7. Duodenum
8. Sphincter muscles
9. Superior mesenteric artery and vein
10. Pancreatic duct
11. Pancreas
12. Common bile duct
13. Common hepatic duct
14. Right and left hepatic ducts

The small intestine

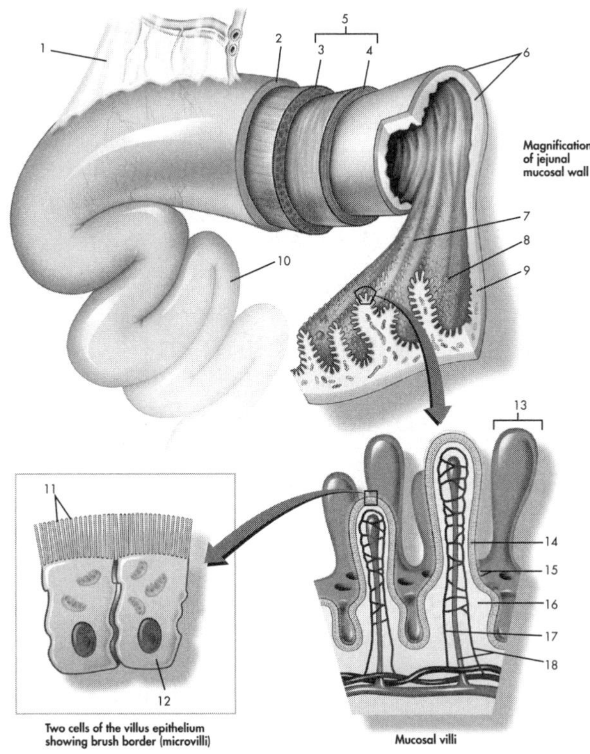

1. Mesentery
2. Serosa
3. Longitudinal muscle
4. Circular muscle
5. Muscularis
6. Submucosa
7. Plica (fold)
8. Lymph nodule
9. Mucosa
10. Segment of jejunum
11. Microvilli
12. Epithelial cell
13. Single villus
14. Mucosa
15. Microvilli
16. Submucosa
17. Lacteal (lymph capillary)
18. Artery and vein

Large intestine

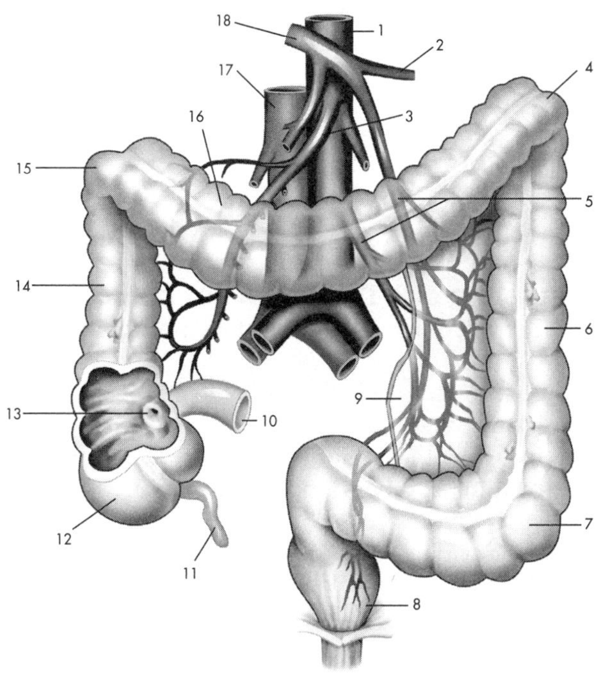

1. Aorta
2. Splenic vein
3. Superior mesenteric artery
4. Splenic (left colic) flexure
5. Inferior mesenteric artery and vein
6. Descending colon
7. Sigmoid colon
8. Rectum
9. Mesentery
10. Ileum
11. Vermiform appendix
12. Cecum
13. Ileocecal valve
14. Ascending colon
15. Hepatic (right colic) flexure
16. Transverse colon
17. Inferior vena cava
18. Portal vein

CHAPTER 16 NUTRITION AND METABOLISM

Fill in the blanks

1. Bile, p. 424
2. Prothrombin, p. 424
3. Fibrinogen, p. 424
4. Iron, p. 424
5. Hepatic portal vein, p. 424

Matching

6. B, p. 427
7. A, p. 424
8. C, p. 427
9. D, p. 428
10. E, p. 428
11. A, p. 424
12. E, p. 428
13. A, p. 428

Circle the one that does not belong

14. Bile (all others refer to carbohydrate metabolism)
15. Amino acids (all others refer to fat metabolism)
16. M (all other refer to vitamins)
17. Iron (all others refer to protein metabolism)
18. Insulin (all others tend to increase blood glucose)
19. Folic acid (all others are minerals)
20. Ascorbic acid (all others refer to the B-complex vitamins)

Circle the correct answer

21. C, p. 428
22. A, p. 430
23. C, p. 431
24. B, p. 431
25. B, p. 432
26. A, p. 432
27. C, p. 432
28. D, p. 432
29. A, p. 431

Unscramble the words

30. Liver
31. Catabolism
32. Amino
33. Pyruvic
34. Evaporation

Applying what you know

35. Weight loss; anorexia nervosa
36. Iron; meat, eggs, vegetables, and legumes
37. She was carbohydrate loading or glycogen loading which allows the muscles to sustain aerobic exercise for up to 50% longer than usual.

38.

C	C	C	B	W	E	F	F	L	J	V	G	G	S
A	T	N	L	W	E	U	O	Z	I	E	L	I	B
R	K	K	P	Z	F	R	I	T	P	O	Y	K	L
B	Q	M	I	N	E	R	A	L	S	J	C	C	P
O	S	S	N	C	X	M	I	D	B	D	O	W	P
H	S	I	Y	O	I	T	X	H	I	N	L	S	N
Y	E	L	N	N	I	K	W	W	D	S	Y	N	S
D	G	O	S	O	W	T	I	U	E	H	S	C	N
R	M	B	Y	T	I	W	C	Z	N	N	I	A	A
A	R	A	Q	W	A	T	B	E	I	G	S	J	M
T	E	T	F	N	I	F	A	E	V	E	W	T	Y
E	V	A	P	O	R	A	T	I	O	N	D	T	E
S	I	C	N	E	S	O	P	I	D	A	O	F	E
H	L	Y	K	I	R	E	B	V	P	A	H	C	J
I	W	E	E	P	A	D	F	T	E	A	R	G	G

Crossword

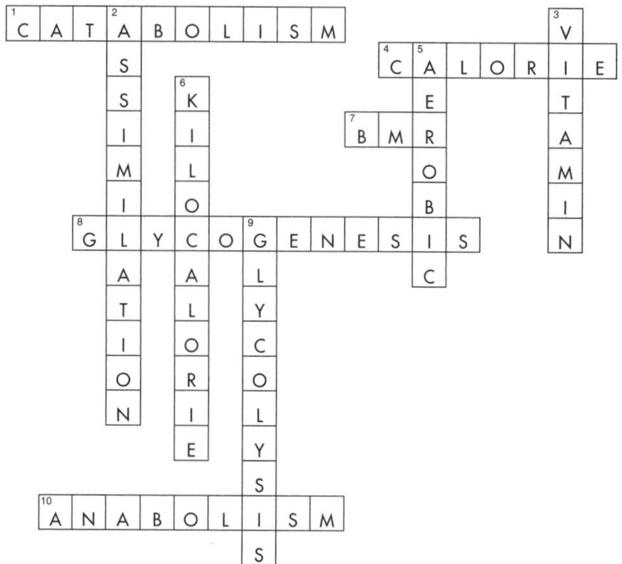

Check your knowledge

Multiple choice

1. B, p. 423
2. A, p. 424
3. C, p. 424
4. C, p. 425
5. B, p. 426
6. B, p. 427
7. A, p. 427
8. A, p. 430
9. B, p. 432
10. D, p. 424

Completion

11. Carbohydrates, p. 424
12. Glycolysis, p. 424
13. Citric acid cycle, p. 424
14. Iodine, p. 430
15. Basal metabolic rate, p. 428
16. Total metabolic rate, p. 430
17. Hypothalamus, p. 431
18. A, p. 429
19. Vegetables, p. 429
20. A, E, D, K, p. 428

CHAPTER 17
URINARY SYSTEM

Multiple choice

1. E, p. 442
2. C, p. 442
3. E, p. 442
4. C, p. 444
5. E, p. 446
6. C, p. 446
7. B, p. 446
8. E, p. 446
9. C, p. 446
10. C, p. 447
11. B, p. 448 (review Chapter 10)
12. D, p. 448

Matching

13. G, p. 442
14. I, p. 448
15. H, p. 440
16. B, p. 442
17. K, p. 442
18. F, p. 442
19. J, p. 442
20. D, p. 442
21. L, p. 442
22. C, p. 442
23. M, p. 450
24. A, p. 442

Indicate which organ is identified

25. B, p. 449
26. C, p. 450
27. A, p. 448
28. B, p. 449
29. C, p. 450
30. C, p. 450
31. A, p. 448
32. C, p. 449
33. B, p. 449
34. A, p. 448
35. B, p. 449

Fill in the blanks

36. Renal colic, p. 449
37. Mucous membrane, p. 448
38. Renal calculi, p. 452
39. Ultrasound, p. 452
40. Reduced, p. 451
41. Renal pelvis, p. 448
42. Semen, p. 450
43. Urinary meatus, p. 450

Fill in the blanks

44. Micturition, p. 451
45. Urination, p. 451
46. Voiding, p. 451
47. Internal urethral, p. 451
48. Exit, p. 451
49. Urethra, p. 451
50. Voluntary, p. 451
51. Emptying reflex, p. 451
52. Urethra, p. 451
53. Retention, p. 451
54. Suppression, p. 451
55. Automatic bladder, p. 451

Unscramble the words

56. Calyx
57. Voiding
58. Papilla
59. Glomerulus
60. Pyramids

Applying what you know

61. Polyuria
62. Residual urine is often the cause of repeated cystitis.
63. A high percentage of catheterized patients develop cystitis, often due to poor aseptic technique when inserting the catheter.

64.

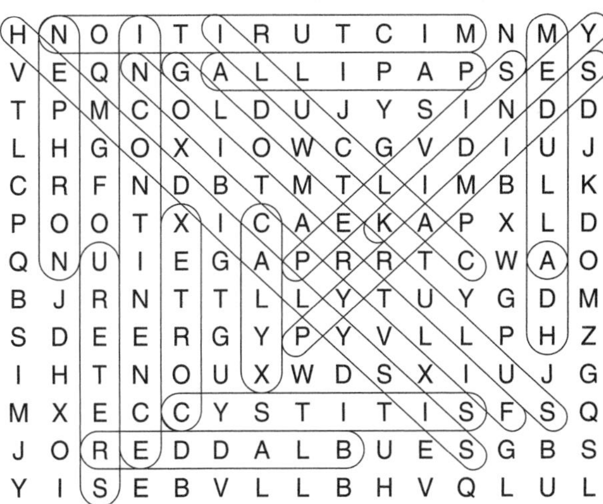

Crossword

		1 M						2 L		3 C	Y	S	T	4 I	T	I	S	
		I		5 T				I		A				N				
		C		R				T		L				C				
		T		I				H		Y				O				
6 G		U		G				O		X			7 A	N	U	R	I	A
L		R		O				T						T				
Y		I		N				R						I				
8 C	A	T	H	E	T	E	R	I	Z	A	T	I	O	N				
O		I						P						E				
S		O						T		9 P				N				
U		N		10 O				O		O				C				
R			11 G	L	O	M	E	R	U	L	U	S		E				
I				I						Y								
A				G						U								
				U						R								
				R						I								
				I						A								
				A														

Check your knowledge

Multiple choice

1. D, p. 441
2. B, p. 442
3. D, p. 444
4. A, p. 446
5. C, p. 446
6. C, p. 452
7. B, p. 448
8. C, p. 448
9. B, p. 449
10. A, p. 446

Matching

11. E, p. 440
12. C, p. 442
13. F, p. 442
14. D, p. 444
15. J, p. 447
16. H, p. 450
17. A, p. 451
18. G, p. 451
19. I, p. 442
20. B, p. 442

Urinary system

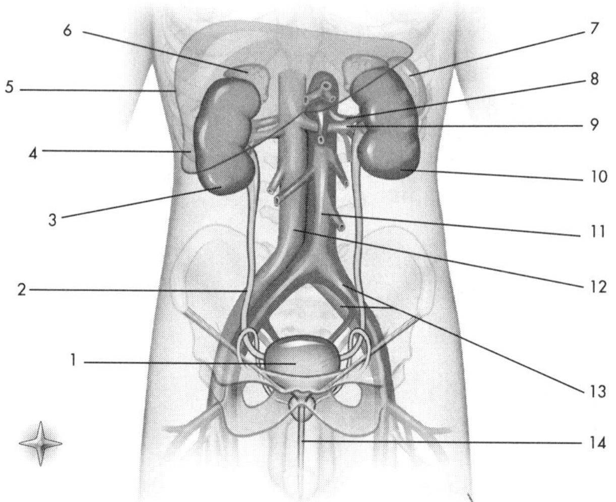

1. Urinary bladder
2. Ureter
3. Right kidney
4. Twelfth rib
5. Liver
6. Adrenal gland
7. Spleen
8. Renal artery
9. Renal vein
10. Left kidney
11. Abdominal aorta
12. Inferior vena cava
13. Common iliac artery and vein
14. Urethra

Kidney

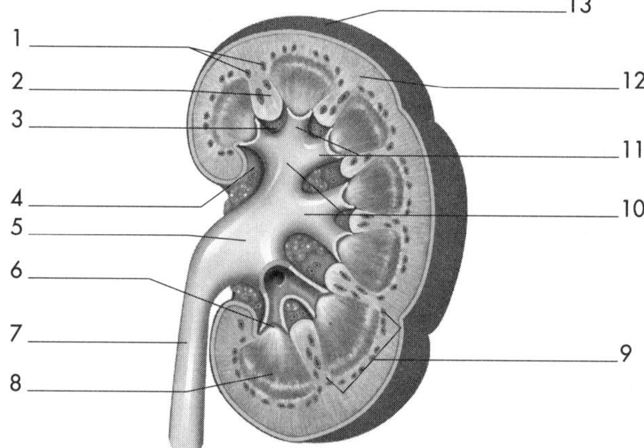

1. Interlobular arteries
2. Renal column
3. Renal sinus
4. Hilum
5. Renal pelvis
6. Renal papilla of pyramid
7. Ureter
8. Medulla
9. Medullary pyramid
10. Major calyces
11. Minor calyces
12. Cortex
13. Capsule (fibrous)

Nephron

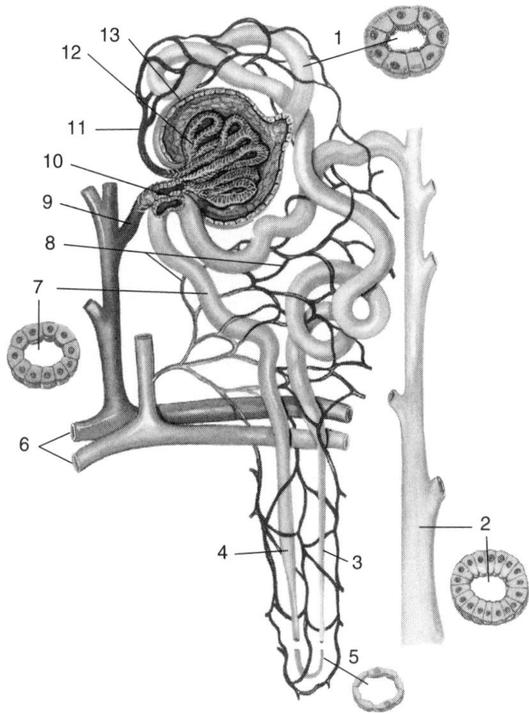

1. Proximal convoluted tubule
2. Collecting tubule
3. Descending limb of Henle's loop
4. Ascending limb of Henle's loop
5. Segment of Henle's loop
6. Artery and vein
7. Distal convoluted tubule
8. Peritubular capillaries
9. Afferent arteriole
10. Juxtaglomerular apparatus
11. Efferent arteriole
12. Glomerulus
13. Bowman's capsule

CHAPTER 18 FLUID AND ELECTROLYTE BALANCE

Circle the correct answer

1. Inside, p. 461
2. Extracellular, p. 461
3. Extracellular, p. 461
4. Lower, p. 460
5. More, p. 460
6. Decline, p. 460
7. Less, p. 460
8. Decreases, p. 460
9. 55%, p. 460
10. Fluid balance, p. 459

Multiple choice

11. A, p. 464
12. D, p. 464
13. A, p. 465
14. A, p. 465
15. C, p. 463
16. E, p. 463
17. D, p. 463
18. D, p. 462
19. C, p. 467
20. B, p. 466
21. D, p. 468
22. E, p. 467
23. B, p. 467
24. B, p. 467
25. B, p. 468
26. E, p. 468

True or false

27. Catabolism, p. 462
28. T
29. T
30. Nonelectrolyte, p. 464
31. T
32. Hypervolemia, p. 466
33. Tubular function, p. 468
34. 2400 ml, p. 463
35. T
36. 100 mEq, p. 467

Fill in the blanks

37. Dehydration, p. 468
38. Decreases, p. 468
39. Decrease, p. 468
40. Overhydration, p. 469
41. Intravenous fluids, p. 469
42. Heart, p. 469

Applying what you know

43. Ms. Titus could not accurately measure water intake created by foods or catabolism, nor could she measure output created by lungs, skin, or the intestines.
44. A careful record of fluid intake and output should be maintained and the patient should be monitored for signs and symptoms of electrolyte and water imbalance.

45.

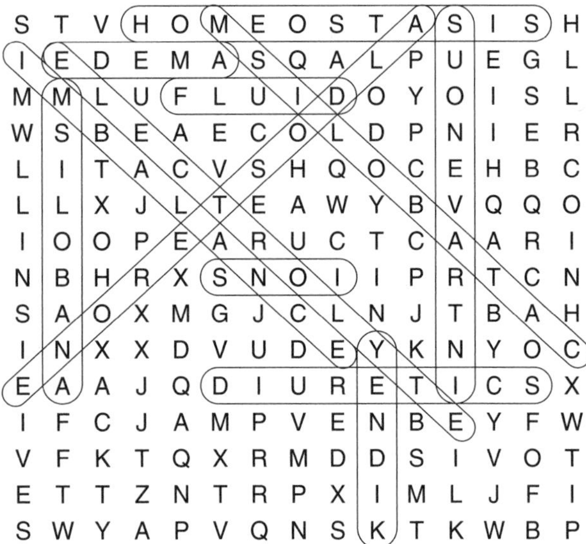

Crossword

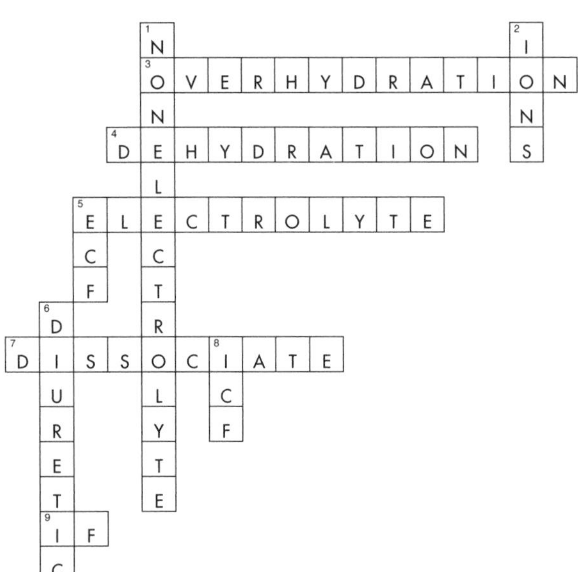

Check your knowledge

Multiple choice

1. A, p. 460
2. D, p. 463
3. D, p. 462
4. C, p. 463
5. A, p. 468
6. B, p. 468
7. D, p. 462
8. A, p. 466
9. A, p. 461
10. D, p. 463

Completion

11. E, p. 461
12. B, p. 461
13. A, p. 464
14. J, p. 464
15. D, p. 468
16. C, p. 459
17. F, p. 468
18. G, p. 468
19. H, p. 469
20. I, p. 467

CHAPTER 19 ACID-BASE BALANCE

Choose the correct term

1. B, p. 476
2. A, p. 476
3. A, p. 476
4. B, p. 476
5. B, p. 476
6. B, p. 476
7. B, p. 476
8. A, p. 476
9. B, p. 476
10. B, p. 476

Multiple Choice

11. E, p. 477
12. E, p. 477
13. A, p. 477
14. E, p. 478
15. C, p. 479
16. D, p. 478
17. C, p. 481
18. B, p. 481
19. D, p. 481
20. E, p. 481
21. E, p. 481

True or false

22. Buffer (instead of heart), p. 477
23. Buffer pairs, p. 477
24. T
25. T
26. Alkalosis, p. 481
27. Kidneys, p. 481
28. T
29. Kidneys, p. 482
30. Lungs, p. 482

Matching

31. E, p. 483
32. G, p. 480
33. F, p. 484
34. A, p. 482
35. I, p. 485
36. B, p. 482
37. H, p. 483
38. C, p. 482
39. D, p. 483
40. J, p. 483

Unscramble the words

41. Fluids
42. Bicarbonate
43. Base
44. Fixed
45. Hydrogen
46. Buffer

Applying what you know

47. Normal saline contains chloride ions, which replace bicarbonate ions and thus relieve the bicarbonate excess which occurs during severe vomiting.
48. Most citrus fruits, although acid-tasting, are fully oxidized during metabolism and have little effect on acid-base balance. Cranberry juice is one of the few exceptions.
49. Milk of magnesia. It is a base. Milk is slightly acidic (see chart, p.).

50.

S	I	S	A	T	S	O	E	M	O	H	P	R	G
E	C	N	A	L	A	B	D	I	U	L	F	E	F
T	S	Y	E	N	D	I	K	W	T	I	K	A	J
Y	D	M	N	D	E	J	W	L	P	T	D	J	I
L	D	N	O	L	H	V	W	O	U	H	D	O	I
O	V	E	R	H	Y	D	R	A	T	I	O	N	S
R	E	I	E	E	D	E	M	A	U	R	O	R	Q
T	L	M	T	C	R	U	L	R	F	S	E	O	Y
C	C	U	S	Z	A	W	E	K	A	T	N	I	X
E	O	Z	O	T	T	T	A	N	A	U	N	M	F
L	F	K	D	P	I	O	I	W	W	Q	L	G	Q
E	N	I	L	C	O	O	H	O	W	S	B	X	S
N	J	X	A	L	N	F	S	U	N	L	J	J	J
O	C	U	V	S	A	L	G	T	I	S	C	Z	X
N	I	Z	L	L	D	Y	X	Q	Q	K	D	C	D

Crossword

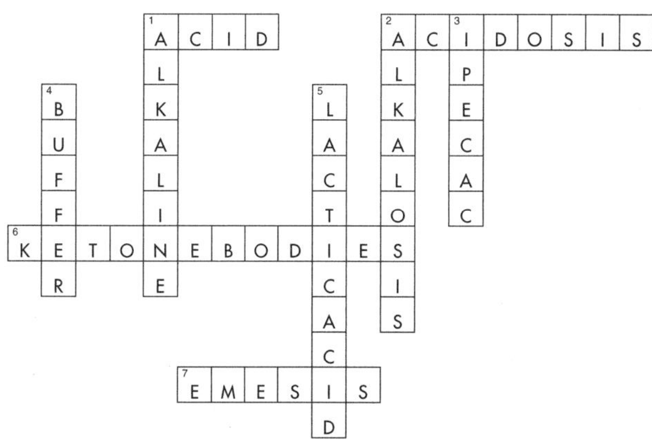

Check your knowledge

Multiple choice

1. A, p. 476
2. C, p. 476
3. A, p. 477
4. D, p. 478
5. A, p. 485
6. D, p. 477
7. D, p. 482
8. D, p. 483
9. D, p. 484
10. A, p. 484

Matching

11. G, p. 477
12. C, p. 476
13. I, p. 477
14. E, p. 478
15. F, p. 478
16. A, p. 480
17. B, p. 477
18. D, p. 481
19. J, p. 483
20. H, p. 483

CHAPTER 20 THE REPRODUCTIVE SYSTEMS

Matching

Group A

1. D, p. 492
2. C, p. 492
3. E, p. 491
4. B, p. 493
5. A, p. 491

Group B

6. C, p. 493
7. A, p. 493

8. D, p. 491
9. B, p. 493
10. E, p. 493

Multiple choice

11. B, p. 494
12. C, p. 494
13. A, p. 495
14. D, p. 498
15. E, p. 494
16. D, p. 495
17. C, p. 495
18. C, p. 495
19. A, p. 495
20. B, p. 498

Fill in the blanks

21. Testes, p. 492
22. Spermatozoa or sperm, p. 495
23. Ovum, p. 491
24. Testosterone, p. 495
25. Interstitial cells, p. 494
26. Masculinizing, p. 497
27. Anabolic, p. 497

Choose the correct term

28. B, p. 497
29. H, p. 499
30. G, p. 499
31. A, p. 497
32. F, p. 498
33. C, p. 498
34. I, p. 498
35. E, p. 498
36. D, p. 499
37. J, p. 499

Matching

38. D, p. 501
39. C, p. 501
40. B, p. 501
41. A, p. 501
42. E, p. 501

Select the correct term

43. A, p. 507
44. B, p. 504
45. A, p. 507
46. B, p. 504
47. A, p. 507
48. A, p. 507
49. A, p. 507
50. B, p. 504

Fill in the blanks

51. Gonads, p. 501
52. Oogenesis, p. 501
53. Meiosis, p. 501
54. One-half or 23, p. 501
55. Fertilization, p.
56. 46, p. 501
57. Estrogen, p. 502
58. Progesterone, p. 502
59. Secondary sexual characteristics, p. 502
60. Menstrual cycle, p. 502
61. Puberty, p. 502

Select the correct term

62. A, p. 505
63. B, p. 504
64. C, p. 505
65. B, p. 504
66. A, p. 503; C, p. 505
67. B, p. 504
68. A, p. 503
69. A, p. 503
70. C, p. 505
71. B, p. 510

Matching

Group A

72. D, p. 505
73. E, p. 505
74. B, p. 505
75. C, p. 505
76. A, p. 505

Group B

77. E, p. 506
78. A, p. 506
79. D, p. 506
80. B, p. 506
81. C, p. 506

True or false

82. Menarche, p. 506
83. One, p. 507
84. 14, p. 507
85. Menstrual period, p. 507
86. T, p. 507
87. Anterior, p. 507

Matching

88. B, p. 508
89. A, p. 507
90. B, p. 508
91. B, p. 508
92. A, p. 510

Unscramble the words

93. Vulva
94. Testes
95. Menses
96. Fimbriae
97. Prepuce
98. Vestibule

Applying what you know

99. Yes. The testes are not only essential organs of reproduction, but are also responsible for the "masculinizing" hormone. Without this hormone, Mr. Belinki will have no desire to reproduce.
100. Sterile—The sperm count may be too low to reproduce but the remaining testicle will produce enough masculinizing hormone to prevent impotency.
101. The uterine tubes are not attached to the ovaries and infections can exit at this area and enter the abdominal cavity.
102. Yes. Yes. Without the hormones from the ovaries to initiate the menstrual cycle, Mrs. Harlan will no longer have a menstrual cycle and can be considered to be in menopause (cessation of menstrual cycle).
103. No. Delceta still will have her ovaries which are the source of her hormones, she will not experience menopause due to this procedure.

104.

M K O V I D U C T S E D H G
S E I R A V O I F U T G L L
I N H Z H M P M K O H I C W
D D V A S D E F E R E N S H
I O A C C I P J V E H Y D S
H M G R R B M N X F G Y I O
C E I O O E Z Y T I C S T E
R T N S T P S D D N O V A D
O R A O U W E B A I J S M Z
T I C M M E Y N E M D L R V
P U A E U D G M I E H I E H
Y M O T C E T A T S O R P B
R P E E R M N E G O R T S E
C O W P E R S I N X K E A P

Crossword

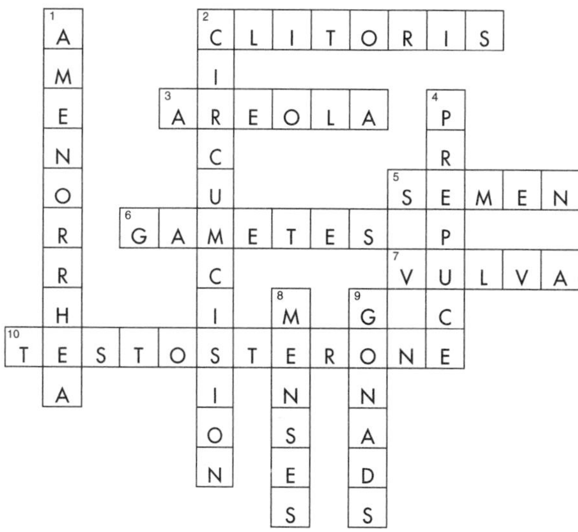

Check your knowledge

Multiple choice

1. A, p. 492
2. D, p. 495
3. D, p. 498
4. C, p. 497
5. C, p. 499
6. A, p. 501
7. B, p. 502
8. C, p. 506
9. A, p. 494
10. D, p. 511

Matching

11. C, p. 491
12. A, p. 495
13. H, p. 495
14. G, p. 499
15. F, p. 499
16. E, p. 510
17. B, p. 495
18. D, p. 506
19. J, p. 505
20. I, p. 506

Male reproductive organs

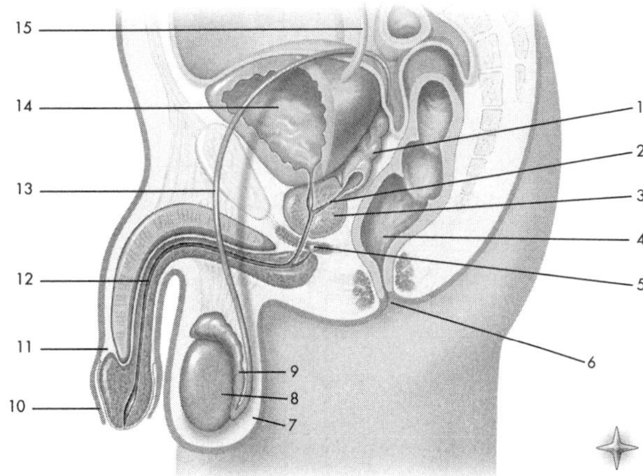

1. Seminal vesicle
2. Ejaculatory duct
3. Prostate gland
4. Rectum
5. Bulbourethral (Cowper's gland)
6. Anus
7. Scrotum
8. Testis
9. Epididymis
10. Foreskin
11. Penis
12. Urethra
13. Ductus deferens
14. Urinary bladder
15. Ureter

Tubules of testis and epididymis

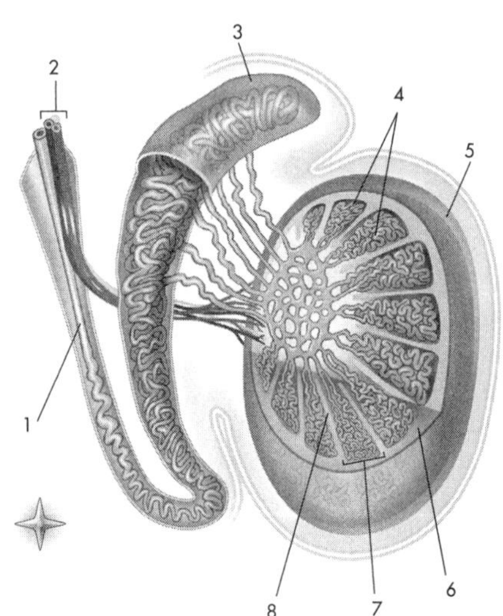

1. Ductus (vas) deferens
2. Nerves and blood vessels in the spermatic cord
3. Epididymis
4. Seminiferous tubules
5. Testis
6. Tunica albuginea
7. Lobule
8. Septum

Vulva

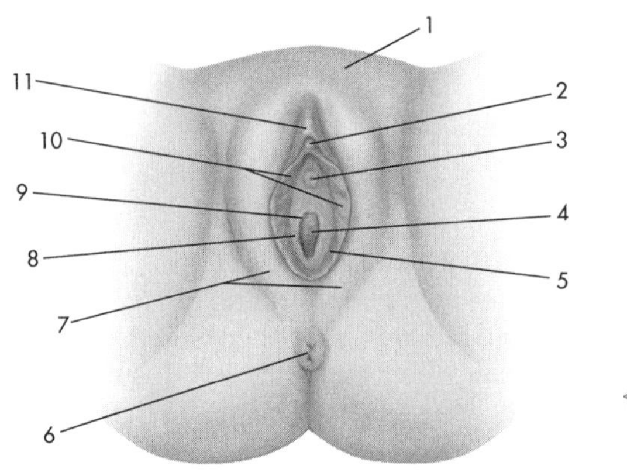

1. Mons pubis
2. Clitoris
3. Orifice of urethra
4. Orifice of vagina
5. Opening of greater vestibular gland
6. Anus
7. Labia majora
8. Vestibule
9. Hymen
10. Labia minora
11. Prepuce

Breast

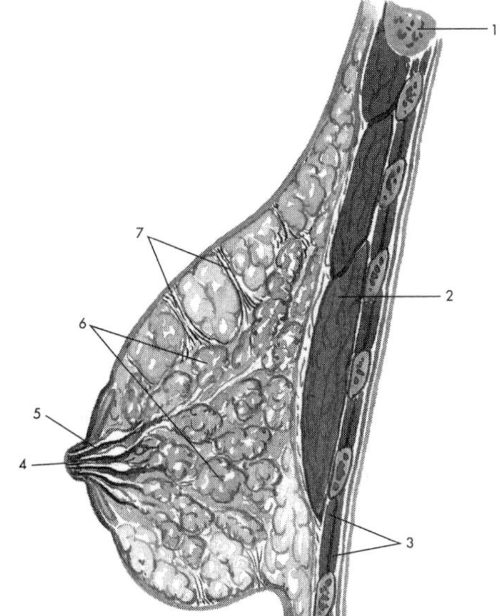

1. Clavicle
2. Pectoralis major muscle
3. Intercostal muscles
4. Nipple pores
5. Lactiferous duct
6. Alveoli
7. Suspensory ligaments of Cooper

Female pelvis

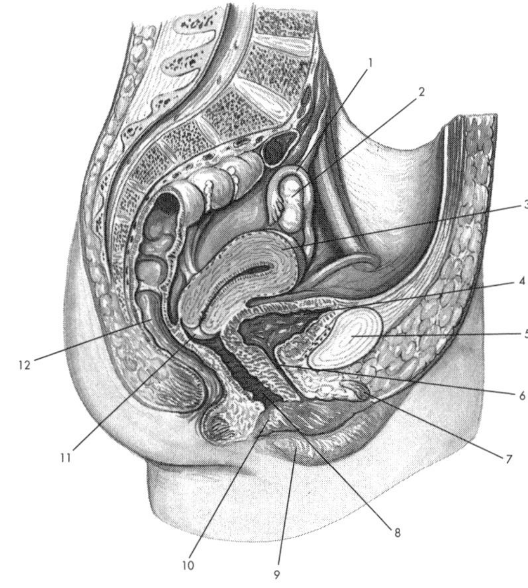

1. Fallopian tube (uterine)
2. Ovary
3. Uterus
4. Urinary bladder
5. Symphysis pubis
6. Urethra
7. Clitoris
8. Vagina
9. Labium majus
10. Labium minus
11. Cervix
12. Rectum

Uterus and adjacent structures

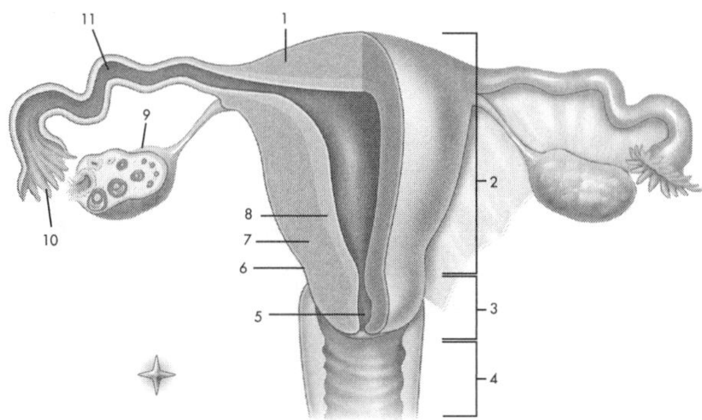

1. Fundus
2. Body of uterus
3. Cervix
4. Vagina
5. Cervical canal
6. Perimetrium
7. Myometrium
8. Endometrium
9. Ovary
10. Fimbriae
11. Uterine (fallopian) tube

CHAPTER 21
GROWTH AND DEVELOPMENT

Fill in the blanks

1. Conception, p. 521
2. Birth, p. 521
3. Embryology, p. 522
4. Oviduct, fallopian tube, or uterine tube, p. 523
5. Zygote, p. 523
6. Morula, p. 523
7. Blastocyst, p. 523
8.. Amniotic cavity, p. 524
9. Chorion, p. 525
10. Placenta, p. 525

Matching

11. G, p. 526
12. F, p. 527
13. C, p. 532
14. B, p. 527
15. A, p. 526
16. H, p. 530
17. E, p. 532
18. D, p. 527
19. I, p. 527
20. J, p. 532

Multiple choice

21. E, p. 531
22. E, p. 533
23. E, p. 534
24. A, p. 534
25. B, p. 534
26. C, p. 534
27. B, p. 534
28. D, p. 534
29. E, p. 534
30. D, p. 534
31. A, p. 534
32. C, p. 534
33. C, p. 534
34. C, p. 534
35. E, p. 534

Matching

36. F, p. 530
37. A, p. 533
38. C, p. 534
39. H, p. 534
40. D, p. 534
41. B, p. 533
42. E, p. 534
43. G, p. 533
44. I, p. 535

Fill in the blanks

45. Lipping, p. 536
46. Osteoarthritis, p. 536
47. Nephron, p. 536
48. Barrel chest, p. 538
49. Atherosclerosis, p. 538
50. Arteriosclerosis, p. 538
51. Hypertension, p. 538
52. Presbyopia, p. 539
53. Cataract, p. 539
54. Glaucoma, p. 539

Unscramble the words

55. Infancy
56. Postnatal
57. Organogenesis
58. Zygote
59. Childhood
60. Fertilization

Applying what you know

61. Normal
62. Only about 40% of the taste buds present at age 30 remain at age 75.
63. A significant loss of hair cells in the organ of Corti causes a serious decline in ability to hear certain frequencies.

64.

```
F T P N O I T A T S E G K F U
Z E P O C S O R A P A L H E A
E O R I L T O H H O C J V J T
C M V T N T I M L N L Z P U O
M A B I I F R M R E D O T C E
H Q C R D L A M E S O D E R M
N N M U Y U I N M F O W G O P
K N V T C O C Z C H H F R C N
H G Y R Y K L T A Y D U C V P
L A T A N T S O P T L U N Q G
Q N K P Y Y S W G A I K E M T
U G P Q N H O Y X Y H O Z B N
I Y T R E B U P L A C E N T A
```

Crossword

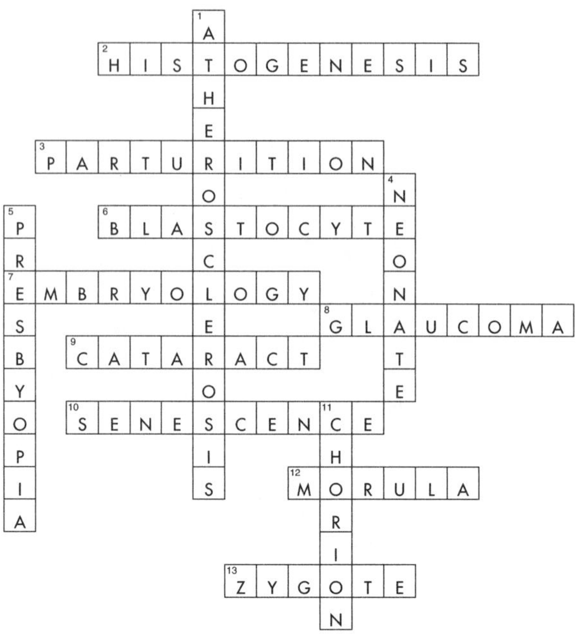

Check your knowledge

Multiple choice

1. C, p. 522
2. D, p. 523
3. D, p. 525
4. A, p. 523
5. D, p. 527
6. D, p. 527
7. C, p. 530
8. A, p. 527
9. C, p. 534
10. B, p. 535

Matching

11. E, p. 522
12. G, p. 523
13. C, p. 527
14. I, p. 535
15. H, p. 560
16. D, p. 532
17. J, p. 536
18. F, p. 539
19. A, p. 535
20. B, p. 533

Fertilization and implantation

1. Ovary
2. Developing follicles
3. Corpus luteum
4. Fimbriae
5. Discharged ovum
6. Spermatozoa
7. First mitosis
8. Uterine (fallopian) tube
9. Divided zygote
10. Morula
11. Blastocyst
12. Implantation

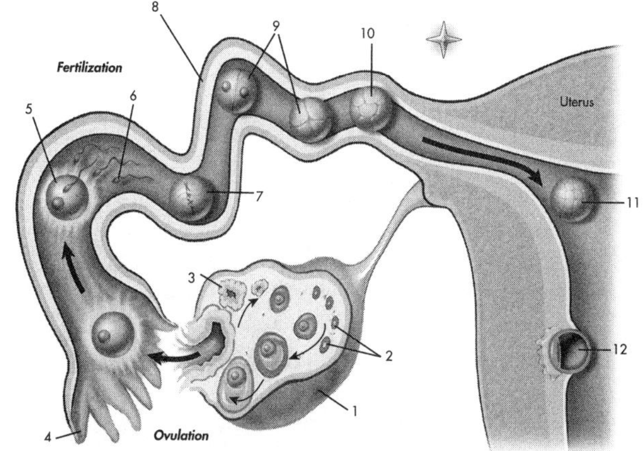